The Mountain
of Youth

The Mountain of Youth

FINDING FITNESS: A GUIDE TO GETTING FITTER, EATING CLEANER, AND LIVING COMPASSIONATELY

Irene Rizzo

ISBN: 1523305541
ISBN 13: 9781523305544
Library of Congress Control Number: 2016900336
CreateSpace Independent Publishing Platform
North Charleston, South Carolina

Internet addresses and telephone numbers given in this book were accurate at the time it went to press.
@2016 by Irene Rizzo

Additional design credits: Cover by Ryden Rizzo, back photo by Jay Sullivan, The Mountain of Youth illustration and graphic by Ryan Patterson and Courtney Feyno
Foreword @ 2016 Neal Bernard, MD

I would like to dedicate *The Mountain of Youth to* the following people:
To my grandson, Landen, it is my hope to make this world a safer, healthier, more compassionate place for him to grow up in.
To my husband, Ron, who encouraged me every step of the way and inspired me to write this book.
To my children—Madison, who helped me get the book started, and Ryden, who created the book cover—and for their love and respect of our lifestyle choices.
To my mother and father for always believing in me and supporting my beliefs throughout my life.
And finally, to all the amazing people I have met along the way that do such great work to help animals and tirelessly enlighten us to the alternatives, which will no doubt be their saving grace.

Table of Contents

Foreword

n our research at the Physicians Committee, we have studied the many ways that nutrition affects our health. Over the years, our research center has welcomed hundreds of volunteers—people aiming to lose weight, tackle diabetes, or free themselves from arthritis, migraines, or other problems, and we have put various diets to the test. In the course of many studies, it has become clear that nutrition is a much more powerful force than most people recognize. Plant-based diets, in particular, have tremendous power to help people lose weight and regain their health. Rather than simply "managing" diabetes, high blood pressure, cholesterol problems, or chronic pain, these healthful diet choices often make these problems disappear.

However, proving that diet changes can help is not enough. People need help bringing this information into their lives. That means breaking old habits and starting new ones. They need help in other ways, too. What kinds of exercise are best? How shall we handle stress? How can we help our families and friends to be healthier, too?

You will find the answers to all of these questions in this book. Irene Rizzo guides you to the mountain of youth in a welcoming and easy to follow way.

This book will help you find a new balance in your life. That means that, along with guidance for the best of nutrition, she will also show you how to put fitness to work. And along with a focus on your personal health, she will also help you focus on the bigger picture: your family and the world you live in.

Especially refreshing is Irene's focus on compassion. She reminds us that our food choices affect much more than our individual health. They also have a profound effect on the welfare of animals and on the health of the earth. In turn, understanding the real consequences of our food choices can help us stay on a healthy path.

I would encourage you to read this book from cover to cover. Every page brings you new insights and new tools.

This book has the power to change your life, and you will love it every step of the way.

Neal D. Barnard, MD, FACC President, Physicians Committee for Responsible Medicine Washington, DC

Acknowledgments

The *Mountain of Youth* would not have been possible without the help and encouragement of many people, especially my husband, Ron Rizzo, who inspired and believed in me. His never-ending love and creative support brought this book to life.

As a mother first and foremost, I would like to thank my children, Madison and Ryden. Their understanding and patience about their mom's strong desire to make the world a healthier place and a safe home for all living creatures is greatly appreciated. Their support and love has helped me to complete *The Mountain of Youth*.

Thank you to my daughter-in-law, Lanette, not only for trusting my choices but also for deciding to become a vegetarian. She also plans on passing it on to my grandson, and for that I am grateful.

Thank you to my mom and dad for their unconditional generosity, for believing in me, and for never trying to change me.

Thank you to my sister, Carol Gordon Ekster, a highly accomplished author of children's books, has set the bar high for me; I hope I make you proud.

A special thank you to Laurie Ann Davis, whose help has been invaluable. Words cannot express my gratitude.

Thank you to Dr. Neal Bernard for taking the time to read "Mountain of Youth" and for writing such an amazing foreword. You have been an inspiration and a guide.

I would like to thank my many clients, who are one of the many reasons I decided to write *The Mountain of Youth*. To all of you, thank you. It is my hope that this will be your guide to help you stay on your path to health and fitness.

To the countless leaders in the vegan community, including Dean Ornish, M.D., Joel Fuhrman, M.D., Caldwell B. Esselstyn, Jr., M.D., T. Colin Campbell, Ph.D., Melanie Joy, Victoria Moran., Joshua Katcher, James Koroni, Gene Baur, Donnie Moss, Jenny Brown Vegan Mos (Ethan and Michael), Gene Stone, Joy Pierson, Bart Potenza, Leanne Mai-ly Hilgart, Kathy Stevens, Liz Dee, Jay Astafa, Jane Velez-Mitchell, Alexander Gray Associates, Jasmine Singer and the New York Coalition for Healthy School Food. Thank you for being an inspiration.

Thank you to the various animal groups who have saved countless animals and fought for their rights. I am proud to stand by your sides and support your work.

To my many teachers, thank you for the gift of fitness and health knowledge. You have helped shape me into the teacher I have become.

Special thanks to all the high-profile celebrities and athletes who bring veganism to the forefront and have helped raise awareness about animals: Jon Stewart and his wife, Tracey McShane; Jerry and Jessica Seinfeld; Ellen DeGeneres and Portia de Rossi; Natalie Portman; Ben Stiller; Johnny Depp; Alec Baldwin; Brad Pitt; Michelle Pfeiffer; Anne Hathaway; Lea Michele; Joaquin Phoenix; Beyoncé and Jay Z; Jennifer Lopez; Christina Applegate; Tobey Maguire; Sara Gilbert; Hilary Swank; Woody Harrelson; Carrie Underwood; Jared Leto; Venus Williams; Carl Lewis; and Mike Tyson.

Introduction

Do you want to know the truth about finding balance and living a compassionate life? As they say, "The truth is hard to swallow."

set out to write *The Mountain of Youth* as a gateway to educate and enlighten others on the many components it takes to find not only a healthy balance in life but also a more compassionate way of living for yourself and others. I want to encourage you to recognize the food on your plate in its original form. Where does it come from, and if you back up the distribution a few steps, would you be happy with the process it takes to get to you? You see, not only can you be a healthier, stronger being, but you can also help preserve the planet and its species. Why not think this way?

It is my passion and drive to help others. For that reason, I decided to put all my years of training, knowledge, and studying to good use. I not only train countless people in my Pilates studio, but as a health coach, I am also constantly sharing information that will help my clients live the healthier, more compassionate, fitter lives they are looking to attain. My clients are also gifts to me. They openly share their struggles while asking so many wonderful questions, which opens the door to a bigger variety of knowledge that I can share with you (you can find a sampling of the questions at the end of the book).

Most would ask, "Why do you have a need to help others and to advocate for animals?" I am a health coach and have been a Pilates instructor with my own studio for over thirty years. It is what I do. It is what I feel in my heart. Being a compassionate human being and animal lover, I do not want to see any living being suffer, and I do know that eating animals will not benefit your health; it will harm instead, and digesting them after they have experienced painful demises will not be beneficial to your emotional state. I do not preach. I practice. Starting with my own life, it has always been my daily goal to maintain a balance. I not only do this for myself, but also for my family, as well as my clients and anyone who touches my life—practicing what I preach and seeing the beneficial results of it. I would also like to think I have helped to assist others to be successful at maintaining balance. When we are successful and happy with our own lives and choices, we can't help but want to share.

I am not telling you to run out and become a vegan (although I really want to shake you so that you can see how passionate and beneficial it would be for your life). I'm saying make some changes, and see how you feel (*then* you can be a vegan). But know that everything you do and put into your body affects you physically and emotionally.

With that said, make it simple. Start with adding more vegetables or fruit to your diet, and exchange those leather shoes or belt for an animal-friendly choice. As a vegan I do all I can to help others understand that they do not have to eat animals in order to be fit. In fact it is the opposite.

In my chapter on compassion, I go into the details of this, and in "Finding Trends," you will see we don't need to wear animals as well. We have so many choices that benefit us and our planet and the beautiful creatures that live among us. As the Vegan Publishers state, "The bodies of others do not belong to us." Animals deserve our compassion. They all have hearts, noses, ears, eyes, and feelings, just like us. So with all that I have learned and lived, why not spread the good news and get others motivated to achieve their goals both physically and mentally while compassionately allowing our fellow creatures to live the lives they deserve?

After a great deal of thinking and devising the best way to approach helping others and sharing what I know, I have come up with the Mountain of Youth, which I lay out for you in the first chapter. It is not as simple as it may look. Remember, it is a process that will take work, but hard work pays off. Nothing good comes easily, as we know, and being busy cannot be an excuse. Make yourself the priority by putting your health at the top of the list. Though I am very busy, I make time for my health, as should you. There is only one you! Finding compassion in your heart will help you. Feeling the joy of exercise will help you in finding your own fitness. I don't want you to give up. I want you to make being healthy a habit that you just can't quit!

So I did all I could to make it an easy climb. It is about taking the steps and finding your footing on your mountain. If you can visualize a rock-climbing wall, picture how you have to use all the parts of your body and mind to achieve the next step to the top. Thinking of the Mountain of Youth will keep you focused and grounded. In rock climbing you are attached to a harness for safety, so see yourself strapping on that harness before you delve into these chapters. It is important for you to think positively as you get ready to find your own balance and climb the Mountain of Youth. Eventually you will become an expert climber. That is why it is all laid out for you step by step in the first chapter.

Finding your balance so you can get to the top of your Mountain of Youth will consist of improving your fitness; having compassion for yourself, others, and animals; being aware of trends and how they can block your progress; discovering healthy alternatives for beauty and joy that will enhance your well-being; and learning from others as I answer their questions.

Ready, get set, go! Find your balance.

Find your healthy balance using the Mountain of Youth. Climb your very own personal mountain, and seek your ultimate life filled with exercise, nutrition, and encouragement. Come with me as we discover a vibrant new you.

Finding Balance

n early 2014 I decided to write this book. As a Pilates instructor and health coach, I have always maintained my professional edge by taking classes, certification seminars and attending health and fitness events. My initial concept was to review the top fitness studios in New York City with my daughter, Madison and create a log for the best of the best. For a year we attended classes at over one hundred different studios (no exaggeration) to put together our thoughts for you.

But something happened along the way while we were collecting our information. I realized that I devoted thirty-plus years to fitness and to the evolution of nutrition and health, and I had something important to say. As I visited all of these fitness studios, I found my "voice" and a strong personal desire to share what fitness is all about in my opinion—that is how The Mountain of Youth was born.

Fitness is not just about taking exercise classes. It is so much more than that. Fitness incorporates everything about life: exercise, conditioning, relationships, health, nutrition, detoxing, compassion, a sense of well-being and joy, plus an appreciation for the beauty in life. Fitness is eating, cleansing, and meditating. Fitness is that energy glow—that happiness that comes alive in you.

Fitness is about balance and finding your balance. But how do you do that? How can you achieve what so many people seek—what I call the Mountain of Youth?

Let's take a look at the how you can begin attaining a Mountain of Youth. Balance is achieved by obtaining overall fitness, which brings together all the components of the Mountain of Youth.

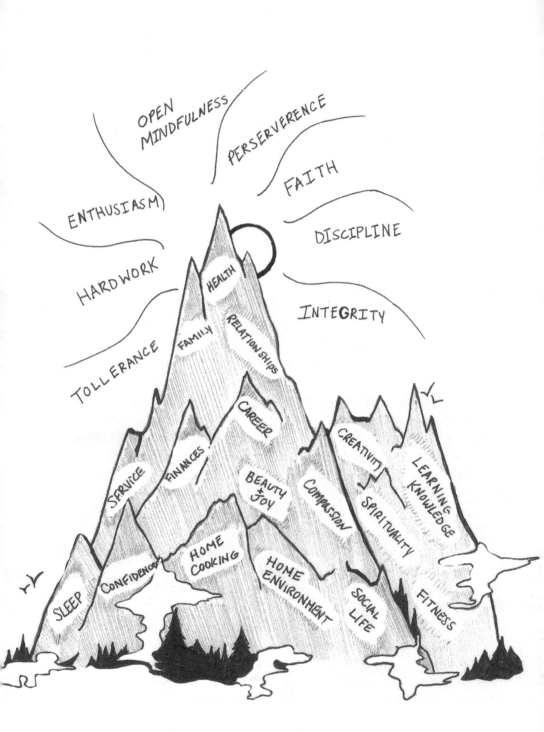

The Mountain of Youth

What Is the Mountain of Youth?

Youth is a metaphor for endless possibility, and the Mountain of Youth is my holistic approach to living. Upon conceiving the Mountain of Youth, I realized the importance of balance in achieving the life of my dreams. Every rock and boulder represents areas of life that could bring to you that youthful feeling and more energy and more happiness than you could ever imagine.

Let's break it down so you can see what a balanced Mountain of Youth looks like.

Health

> We believe if a [plant-based] diet came in a pill, it would
> be heralded on the front pages of newspapers and
> magazines around the world for its effectiveness.
> —ALONA PULDE, MD, AND MATTHEW LEDERMAN, MD

Health is eating whole foods, hydrating your body, and exercising. You can find "health" through simple life changes, like balancing the body with alkaline food and water. Alkaline food is lush green plants, fruits, and vegetables and that should be 70–80 percent of your diet. (See chart at the end of the chapter) Lets examine any fish aquarium for example; the fish cannot survive if the water isn't properly pH balanced. Similarly, your body needs a balanced PH, and temperature for optimal survival. If you body temperature is up, you feel sick, and if your diet isn't balanced with a variety of vegetables and fruits which provide the necessary alkaline balance to your body's chemistry you will also get sick. Science proves that disease cannot breed in an alkaline environment.

Every meal should include a large portion of healthy greens to aid in maintaining proper pH levels and total digestion. Simply stated by Tony Robbins on this subject "Go Green" When you feel good which will be a result of incorporating these wonderful habits into your life, you will notice the difference. If you have your health, you have the foundation for everything you will need to build a Mountain of Youth

Family

> Family is the most important thing in the world.
> —PRINCESS DIANA

My family is the center of my life. It's where our lives begin and where we first learn about love, acceptance, and loyalty. Our parents can be our role models; we look up to them and ingest everything they do. Family isn't always blood; it's the people in your life who love you no matter what and will do anything for you.

I love the symbol of the family tree, since we all come from the same root but branch out on our own. For me I feel my family in my heart and think of them as the most important part of my mountain.

They are all a blessing in my life.

Relationships

Surround yourself with positive, loving, and supportive people. There are some people whom we can't always choose. Our families are handpicked for us, and the healthiest thing to do is to make these relationships work for us. Communication is key to all relationships, whether with family, coworkers, lovers, children, and so forth. They do take work. You can't expect them to grow or change without communication; just like a flower, without water they will not grow—they will die. Find the love and support that suit you best. Balance out togetherness and aloneness. Everyone has his or her own idea of what relationships should be. What it comes down to is discovering ones that make you feel good.

Remember too that a variety of physical touch is crucial to our well being and relationships. It could be as simple as hugging or laying your hand on someone's shoulder or more expansive, such as giving a massage. Touch is needed for relationship survival and self-preservation. Don't settle for less.

Social Life

New studies found that in terms of long life, strong ties with family and friends are as important as losing weight if you are obese, or getting active if you are sedentary.

Nurture existing relationships, get together with family, take a walk with a friend or reach out to a neighbor, ask a colleague to lunch, get to know others or get involved in your community and most importantly be supportive because providing support is more rewarding than receiving support.

Beauty and Joy

Find the beauty and joy in all that's around you. Take the time to be grateful for all you have. Notice nature, the beauty of it, and the joy it brings. Find the beauty in people, animals, and your environment. It's about taking a moment to breathe through quiet times and meditation.

It's also about taking the time to know what looks best on you, getting the right haircut, and keeping yourself well groomed. You're only as old as you think you are. I'm not saying at sixty or seventy you're going to look and feel like you're twenty, but it's important to make the time to look your best. It's amazing how great you can feel when you make the effort (see the chapter "Finding Beauty and Joy").

Spirituality

It doesn't have to be organized religion, although it can be. For me it is kindness, and being grateful for my life, and feeling a sense of a higher power, like in meditation, or exploring nature and being open minded that having faith, it all works out. Find a practice that resonates for you. You will find yourself feeling nourished in profound ways when you discover your connection.

Compassion

We all say we are compassionate beings, but we need to spread this compassion as awareness to all living things. It goes well beyond "us" because by being compassionately aware we could possibly save the planet for our future generations.   Plant-based diets are a large part of what feeds into effortless youth and earth saving results.

Creativity

I hear this all the time: "I don't have a creative bone in my body." Creativity comes in all forms—art, music, dance, and more. You are probably more creative than you think you are. Look within. Cooking is creative, as is gardening or organizing a party or event. There is a great book by Julia Cameron called *The Artist's Way* that will open a world of creative thoughts and ideas if you are curious to expand. Or just simply write in a journal your thoughts and feelings, and your creative energy will grow with each new day. See a live show; visit a museum or art gallery. Get back to nature, and go on a hike. It will clear your mind and open up your creativity. Meditation, relaxation, and guided imagery are great tools. There are many apps you can download to help you with this, or venture out and take a meditation workshop. All these things will help enhance your creative life. Now, go and get creative!

Finances
Healthy finances and a healthy lifestyle go hand in hand. As you turn good habits into a passion, your finances will follow.

Career
Hopefully you are in a career that you love, but if not, look for the hidden passions in what you do and be open to new opportunity.

Learning
To learn is to grow. Nourish your brain with knowledge, and achieve a healthier you. Take workshops or classes that expand your mind. You can self-educate by reading, writing, and spending time with others who possess knowledge you would not otherwise be exposed to.

Home Cooking
Everybody is always so busy and grabbing meals on the go. If you just make half of your meals at home, you will reap the health benefits. Knowing where your food comes from and how it's prepared can make all the difference in the way you feel and look. And home cooking doesn't have to be complicated; it is food you make yourself, food where you know what the ingredients are, and food that's natural and simple. Always cook fresh with organic ingredients whenever possible and allow for lots of fruits and vegetables. Not only will treating yourself to home cooking keep you healthier, but it will also bring on positive feelings when you are caring for yourself and nourishing your body.

Home Environment

When your space at home feels disorganized, you will feel disorganized. Create a space that makes you feel good and safe.

Physical Activity and Intelligent Movement

The Mountain of Youth is also about finding the form of exercise you most enjoy. Mine is Pilates (we'll talk about my passion for Pilates in a later chapter!). Regular exercise is the number-one detox. We are meant to move or we die.

Confidence

Confidence is within all of us, or simply put, it is the "belief in you." I know this all to well from personal experience. My confidence falters at times, but I am lucky that I have the love and support from family so I can be free to listen to my inner voice. It is essential to your well being to be confident, as it may feel like it comes in waves. You will feel more confident on some days, but know that you have the tools to accomplish anything. Start simply with squashing those negative thoughts by acquiring a posture that you recognize as confident. I dare you to stand up tall and put a big smile on your face and then be sad, your physiology will over ride the thoughts that do not serve you well.

Sleep

Don't forget sleep, which is also very important to the Mountain of Youth. Your body can't have the energy you need if you're not sleeping, hydrating, or moving. When your body likes something, it lets you know! It tells you if it's not feeling good. If you're tired, there's something wrong. For example, your body consistently will tell you if you're missing nutrition or need something else, like sleep or exercise. And if you're listening to it, you'll see long-term health benefits.

Service

> The best way to find you is to lose yourself in the service of others.
>
> —GANDHI

Giving without any expectations is the best way of receiving. How often do you ask, "Can I help you?"

Do you get it?

What does your optimal Mountain of Youth look like?

For me, it's spending time with family; it's eating healthy and compassionately; it's exercising intelligently; it's helping other people achieve their goals; it's meditating and taking a moment to breathe; it's hydrating my body and getting enough sleep.

It is also living and breathing joy. I actively pursue my passions. One is helping people to understand that everything they do affects how they think. How they think affects how they feel. How they feel gives them the drive and desire to become the best people they can be. This is what I call intelligent movement—moving toward the achievement of balance in your physique, your emotions, and your life choices.

When you get to the top of your Mountain of Youth, you can enjoy each ray of sunshine you have created to achieve your personal balance for a healthier you.

Alkaline Foods

Vegetables:

Asparagus
Broccoli
Chili
Capsicum/Pepper
Zucchini
Dandelion
Snow peas
Green Beans
String Beans
Runner Beans
Spinach
Kale
Wakame
Kelp
Collards
Chives
Endive
Chard
Cabbage

Coriander
Basil
Brussels Sprouts
Cauliflower
Carrot
Beetroot
Eggplant
Garlic
Onion
Parsley
Celery
Cucumber
Watercress
Lettuce
Peas
Broad Beans
New Potato
Pumpkin Radish
Sweet Potato

Fruit:

Avocado
Tomato
Lemon
Lime
Grapefruit
Coconut

Breads:

Sprouted Bread
Sprouted Wraps
Gluten/Yeast Free
Breads/Wraps

Oils:

Avocado Oil
Coconut Oil
Flax Oil
Olive Oil

Grains and Beans:

Amaranth
Buckwheat
Brown Rice
Chia/Salba
Kamut
Millet
Quinoa
Spelt
Lentils
Lima Beans
Mung Beans
Navy Beans
Pinto Beans
Red Beans
Soy Beans
White Beans

Nuts and Seeds:

Almonds
Coconut
Flax Seeds
Pumpkin Seeds
Sesame Seeds
Sunflower Seeds

Grasses:

Wheatgrass
Barley Grass
Dog Grass
Shave Grass
Oat Grass

Sprouts:

Soy Sprouts
Alfalfa Sprouts
Amaranth Sprouts
Broccoli Sprouts
Fenugreek Sprouts
Mung Bean Sprouts
Quinoa Sprouts
Radish Sprouts
Spelt Sprouts

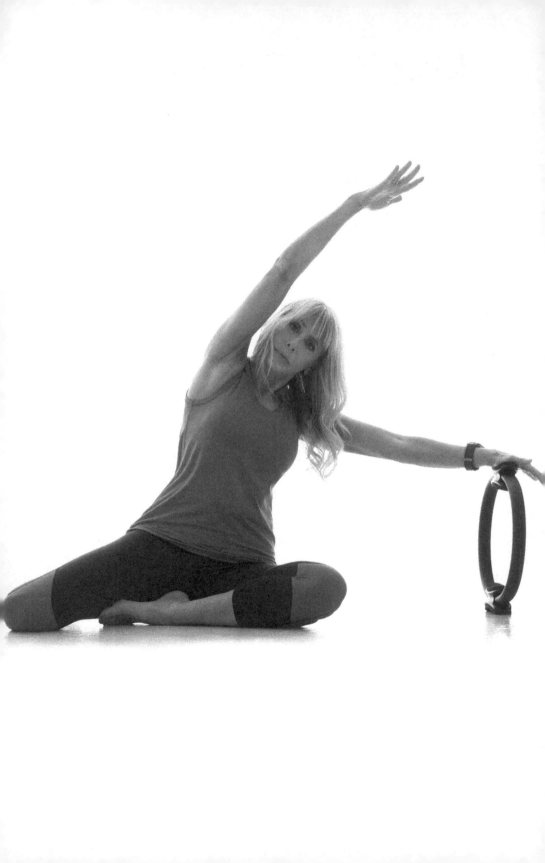

Intelligent Movement

To me, if life boils down to one thing, it's
movement. To live is to keep moving.
—Jerry Seinfeld

Nothing is more revealing than movement.
—Martha Graham

ave you ever felt a painful muscle twinge during exercise? What do you do when that happens? Do you ignore the pain and keep going with your routine to keep up with the girl or guy next to you? Or do you listen to your body, stop, and modify the intensity of your workout?

If you do the latter, you've just practiced what I call intelligent movement. That little twinge is telling you something. But you have to listen to it.

Intelligent movement is another one of my life's passions. Why is it so important to me? Well, as a fitness instructor and health coach with more than three decades of experience, I've found that intelligent movement is a strong foundation to a person's quest for balance in life.

In short, intelligent movement is the source of the Mountain of Youth. Movement is amazing. It is the best medicine you can ever ask for, along with a healthy diet.

Think about it. Your body is so intelligent! If something is bothering you, either during exercise or even during the course of your day, it's the start of something. And the way we find our center—our balance—is by listening and asking ourselves, "What makes me feel happy and good? If I feel bad, why is that?"

If you eat the right food, your body feels good. If you exercise in the right way, your body moves better. You just have to put it all together and listen.

Intelligent people listen.

And intelligent people seek balance. We all have it in us. Why not utilize it?

Helping You to Achieve Balance

When I work with my clients, I tell them, "I'm not in your body. You have to tell me what's going on. Listen to what's going on, and tell me. I will help you get to that next level."

So think of me as your personal coach, helping *you* to that next level. I've been keeping people motived to stay fit and healthy for twenty-five years. I owned and operated a studio in New York City and have trained many high-profile clients. I now specialize in the techniques of Joseph Pilates and holistic health coaching and have uniquely integrated these techniques into my own holistic approach to health. I hold four top certifications for personal training, nutrition, strength, and the Pilates method. (Those certifications are with Physical Mind, ACE, and Integrated Nutrition.)

The Pilates method is a premier form of body conditioning, emphasizing body alignment and correct breathing. The method uses the abdomen, lower back, and hips as a power center, enabling the rest of the body to move freely. It emphasizes performing the exercises in a precise manner while helping you progress at your own individual rate. It is the foundation of what intelligent movement is all about.

Joseph Pilates is such an inspiration to me! His determination to restore the health and vitality of others has fueled my own desire to help people in their quests for balance.

Joseph once said, "The acquirement and enjoyment of physical well-being, mental calm and spiritual peace are priceless to their possessors." And achieving that is exactly why I wrote this book for you.

My goal is not only to give you guidance to help you find fitness through active balance, but also to give you guidelines for the other aspects of your life—for intelligently moving toward your balance and achieving that ideal Mountain of Youth.

We'll discuss my personal views on why the vegan lifestyle is so valuable (both for you and for the planet), what fitness really is, how to incorporate fitness into a fun lifestyle (massages, great food, vegan treats, shopping for new clothes for the new you, manicures—yes, for you guys too! —and blowouts for the ladies after a workout are wonderful gifts to yourself!) as well as how to feel good and joyful about who you are and the beauty that surrounds you.

I also hope that by the time you finish reading, you'll have a firm grasp on what it takes to find fitness, wholeness, beauty, joy, and balance.

"It is the mind itself which builds the body," Joseph Pilates once said.

Let's start building together.

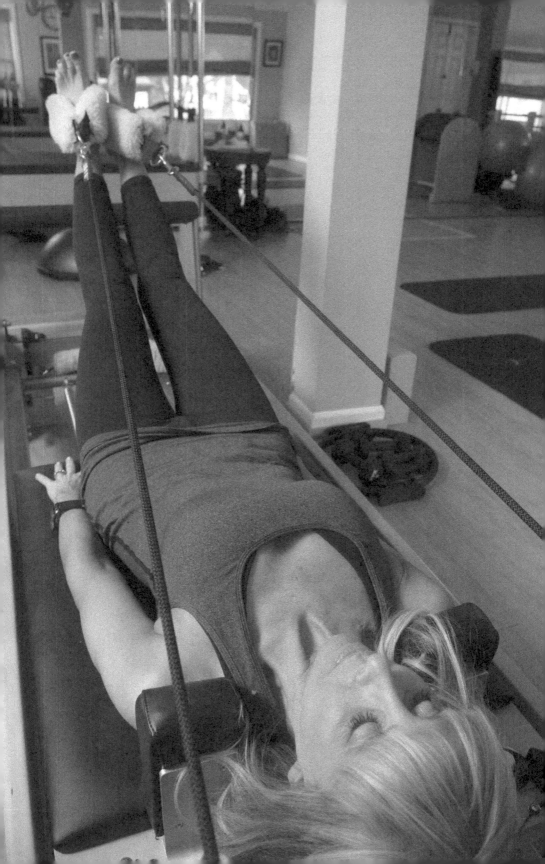

Finding Pilates

Physical fitness is the first requisite of happiness.

If your spine is inflexibly stiff at 30, you are old. If it
is completely flexible at 60, you are young.
—JOSEPH PILATES

When I meet people and tell them I'm a Pilates instructor, they say, "What is Pilates? Is that like yoga?"

Most people really don't understand it, and when I was first introduced to it in my twenties, I didn't either.

I love Pilates.

No, really.

When I say, "I love Pilates," I really mean that I am very passionate about the Pilates technique and believe the method will keep your body young.

The funny thing about Pilates is that it works every small muscle as well as the large muscle groups, where the challenge and focus is on the "Powerhouse". Joseph Pilates created the term Powerhouse to describe the section of the body starting from the bottom of the ribs down to the top of the hips and all the way to the bottom of the pelvis. This is where Pilates gets is reputation for being an unbelievable core workout.

But here's the sweet thing about a lot of the exercises: you're not working against gravity. You're lying down! It is hard, but at the same time, the equipment embraces and supports you, helping you to get through all the exercises. Please do not be fooled, if you feel that the exercises are easy you are probably not doing them correctly.

Anyone from a beginner on up can benefit from Pilates, the elite athlete or the person recovering from an injury or anyone looking to get to the next level of fitness and flexibility. This approach to fitness can be as difficult or as easy as you want it to be. You will feel the improvement in your body before you see the results. You can though expect to see a different reflection of yourself in the mirror, even if you only work out two to three times per week. I've seen people totally change the way they look and feel in as few as ten sessions of training. Keep in mind that a perfect body only exists in "Photoshop", so if you set your mind on feeling good, vibrant and healthy you will be pleasantly surprised with the outcome. Every celebrity, super model, athlete and even sports teams have incorporated Pilates into their routines.

As a student of this discipline, you'll find that Pilates will lengthen, strengthen, and tone your body. Pilates is meant to help you build core strength—front and back. It keeps your spine flexible and allows you to move freely through your various tasks of the day, as your range of motion will improve. You'll even notice you are breathing more deeply and filling your body with needed oxygen. And it's always nice when your waistband starts to loosen, isn't it? That's another benefit you'll see. Pilates is about changing your body from the inside out, as your joints will become more flexible and your abdomen will begin to flatten. I have noticed that when I leave a great Pilates session, I stand taller and feel more alive. No one ever gets tired of that feeling!

What Is Pilates?

Pilates (pronounced pill-*ah*-tees, not pie-lates) is named after its creator, Joseph Pilates, who once said, "A man is as young as his spinal column." This is the core of his groundbreaking approach to exercise that revolutionized the world of fitness and health.

He was born in 1880 and was a sickly child. As a young man, he became passionate about physical fitness as a way to improve his health and appearance. He studied and practiced gymnastics, boxing, karate, and yoga. He even performed in circuses! He combined the philosophies of East meets West before anybody else.

In World War I, he was interned at a prison camp in England. During his imprisonment Mr. Pilates became stronger, using anything around him to exercise, such as springs from the beds or a chair. He began to teach everyone in prison camp his methods. Pretty soon everyone was getting stronger and healthier. He was a genius and studied the body's physiology until he knew it inside out.

After the war, around 1925, Mr. Pilates immigrated to the United States and met his wife, Clara, on the ship voyage to his new country. After arriving, he opened his first studio in New York City. Today his method has become wildly popular.

Six Principles of Pilates

There are six basic principles of Pilates:

1. Concentration: By focusing on your body awareness, you establish better connection with your body, and you gain more benefits from your workouts. It's better to do each exercise slowly and precisely than with incorrect form or posture.
2. Centering: By paying attention to the muscles of the core (the Pilates Powerhouse), you will help all of your body's muscle function and develop more efficiently.
3. Control: In Pilates, slow and steady wins the race. Control, rather than intensity or repetition, is key to performing the exercises correctly. All movements should be performed with precision to gain the maximum benefits.
4. Breathing: Controlling your breath with deep exhalations as you perform each exercise helps activate your muscles and keep you focused.
5. Precision: Practice makes perfect. Proper form is essential to ensure you gain the most benefit and keep your body healthy.
6. Flow: Each motion should be smooth and graceful. Try to create the grace of a dancer or a gymnast in your practice.

(See http://pilates.about.com/od/whatispilates/a/Principles.htm for more information.)

Mr. Pilates once wrote, "To achieve the highest accomplishments within the scope of our capabilities in all walks of life, we must constantly strive to acquire strong, healthy bodies and develop our minds to the limits of our ability." I find myself thinking about the mind and body connection almost every day.

I enjoy watching films of Mr. Pilates, who had a great daily routine. One of my favorite scenes in the archival footage is his demonstration of the first few moments of his morning. He attached springs to his bed. When he woke, he grabbed onto these springs to do an exercise called the Pilates hundreds. This involves raising your torso and legs into a V, reaching forward with your straightened arms, and pumping your hands up and down one hundred times. This warm-up exercise strengthens your core abdominal muscles and revs up your circulation, getting everything moving.

I try to emulate Mr. Pilates in the same way. Even when I'm traveling on vacation, the first thing I do when I wake up in my hotel room is to get out of bed, lie down on the floor, and do the hundreds just like he did. It makes me feel so energized and ready to start the day!

In the Pilates community, many instructors feel it is necessary to teach these methods to the letter, just as Mr. Pilates taught them. However, Mr. Pilates was such a forward thinker in his time. It is my belief that his method would evolve if he were alive today. I do think Mr. Pilates would stay true to his classical principles. But I also think exercise equipment has improved. These advancements would naturally lead to new approaches and the blending of his various techniques. I feel privileged to expand on his ideas.

The Class That is Right for You

So if you came to one of my Pilates classes, what would you find me teaching?

I prefer what we call the classical Pilates workout—one that sticks to the original ideals that Mr. Pilates first established but also accommodates each student's needs and abilities. As a longtime teacher who has taken lessons and workshops with all of the top teachers and studios, I find that you can't help but give Pilates your own flavor and your own individual stamp so that you can accommodate the person who is standing in front of you.

A good instructor is one who can keep you moving and explain the exercise simultaneously. By the end of the class, you should feel like you've worked out. You should feel good. When you walk out of the studio, you'll feel that extra something special—you'll feel taller; you'll be standing better with better posture. You should feel overall that your breathing is connected to your physique. You'll feel more confident, because you've been moving your body, challenging it in new ways. You have put yourself through a wonderful workout! You'll walk back out into the world, taking all of that goodness with you. If you've ever had a great fitness session like that, you know exactly what I'm talking about.

There is a general agreement in the Pilates community that after ten training sessions, you should feel a physical difference in your body, but after twenty sessions, you should *see* the difference. As a result, I recommend to clients that they sign up for twenty, because I know they'll be happy with the results as it doesn't take that long to see the change!

I recommend you book a class at what I would deem a forward-thinking studio. And how do you find one? My experience is that the studios that are the busiest are the ones that have come up with the best ways to work your body the hardest. Look for those where you'll have a tough time booking a spot. It's worth the extra effort—trust me.

It's really best to take private lessons so that you are instructed about the correct form of Pilates exercises and how to do them properly. Although I find that Pilates is extremely safe, it's easier to ask a teacher for guidance in a private lesson than in a large class setting. As in anything else, you can always get hurt. It's worth it to have one-on-one instruction that will be tailored to your body and your needs.

My Healing Journey

I found Pilates first at age twenty-nine, and then I found it again years later.

When I was first introduced to Pilates, I didn't know what it was, and I didn't understand all of the good it could do. I was teaching it but only scratching the surface of this glacier. It was 1986, and I opened my first business and christened it Irene's Fitness Studio. I incorporated aerobics and exercises inspired by Jane Fonda.

When I first started training to become an exercise instructor, my teachers used the Pilates style of exercise. But I had no idea it was called Pilates, and even they did not use that word for it. They called it Contrology, a word Mr. Pilates also used to describe his approach. I thought it was the weirdest exercise! I used it in my repertoire, but it didn't make sense to me. Lie on the floor, and pump your arms? What was that all about? I didn't have a deep understanding of it and didn't fully appreciate it.

A dozen years later, in 1998, I was now a mom and found myself facing a health crisis. I woke up one morning and had trouble moving. I had two herniated discs. I saw eleven different neurologists for help, and they all told me that if I didn't have surgery, I would eventually be paralyzed on the left side of my body.

How had this happened? My theory is that I'd had a couple of bad falls. I used to go horseback riding, and I'd also had bad falls while rollerblading and ice-skating. I may have been injured for a while and did something unknowingly to trigger it.

At the time, I had a high amount of stress in my life, which was another contributing factor. I tell my clients all of the time that sometimes you have underlying physical issues that are not aggravated until you face things in your life that are stressful. We abuse our bodies all the time. Combine that with gravity and age, and you never know when something like this will strike.

My children, a son and a daughter, were young. Because of the injury, I couldn't even drive a car and had to get someone else to drive them to school!

I went to an osteopathic doctor, who encouraged me to exercise. And you may find this hard to believe, but I decided that maybe it was time to get back into teaching fitness and going for my certification. But, I asked myself, in what?

I met a woman who was teaching Pilates, and she asked if I wanted to teach it with her. She said she'd train me. I agreed. Three months later, between working with her and the osteopathic doctor, I had healed. I never needed the surgery or experienced serious pain after that. Through Pilates I was able to gain the flexibility and strength I needed to heal. .

This system saved my life. The energy I get from doing just a little every day is wonderful. On average I do Pilates for a half hour to an hour about six times per week. I also add another form of exercise—aerobics or walking—each day. And on the week-ends, I try to take other people's classes (Pilates or another form of exercise, like yoga).

You should try to do Pilates at least twice per week, and you should do something for your body every single day. If Pilates is your only form of exercise, try to do it four times per week, and incorporate walking on the in-between days. My opinion is that only elite athletes can afford to do Pilates once a week. Everyone else should be doing it much more frequently.

I have found that Mr. Pilates believed in many of the practices in which I strongly believe, from dry brushing to cleaning out your sinuses. I also admire many of the in-structors who carry on his work, all doing it with their own twists, even if they all think they present it the same way.

Pilates brought me back to myself, and it can do the same for you if you give it a try.

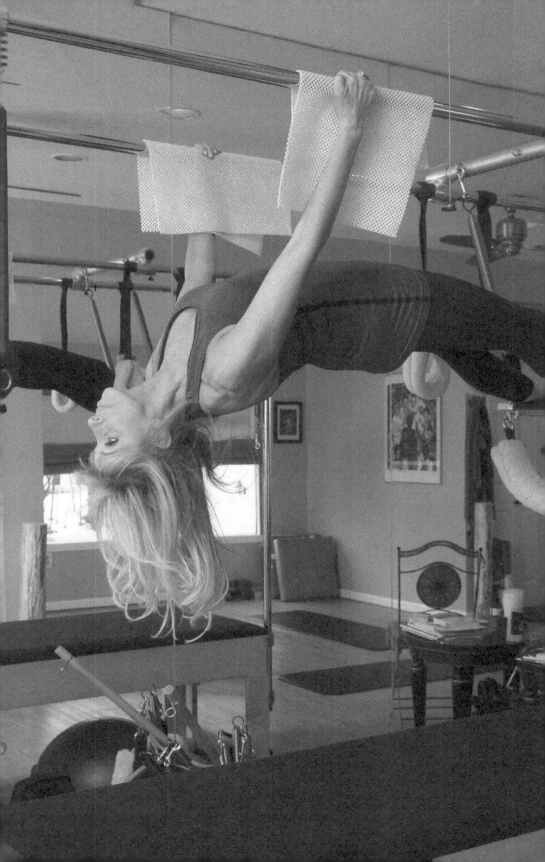

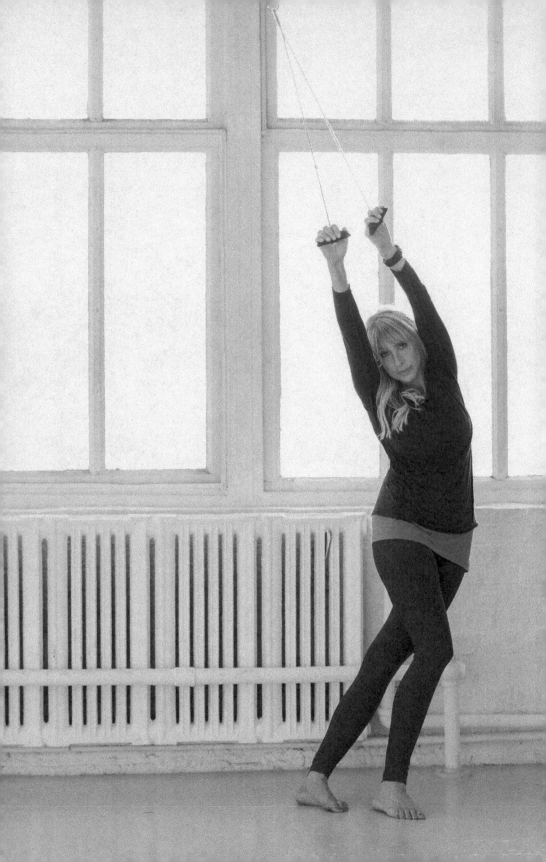

Finding Trends

Trends will come and go. Loving yourself, being who
you are and being OK with all of it, that is forever. Self-
compassion is a priceless gift you give yourself.
—COACHINGBYCODIE

Trends come and go in the worlds of fashion, home décor, and even the conjoined universes of fitness and nutrition.

I've been entrenched in the fitness industry since the 1980s, so I can safely say I've seen a lot of trends. And I watch them with great interest, because the fitness trend of the day ultimately affects people's health—not just their physiques in the short term but, as they age, their futures in the big picture.

While it's fun to be part of the latest and greatest fitness regimen, it also pays to be aware of how a new fad may affect your overall health and well -being.

In this chapter I'd like to walk you through how I've seen fitness trends change over the years—the good, the bad, and the ugly. We'll also talk about current fitness trends and the positives and negatives they may bring to your life.

At the end of the day, the most important thing I want you to remember is that when finding trends, find those that improve and enhance your life—not those that can potentially take away from it.

My Career Started with Jane Fonda's Workout

When I first started in my career as a fitness coach in the 1980s, there weren't many fitness classes. They were a rarity, and now they're everywhere, popping up every place you look. You should have no problem finding a variety of classes in your area.

Currently there is an explosion of "boutique" studios, each of which provides its own flavor of unique classes.

We've come a long way with fitness trends. The beginning of my career saw the trend of Jane Fonda and high-impact aerobics. In fact, at the time Jane's methods became popular, I went to California and exercised for six weeks at her studio to learn her approach. "No pain, no gain" was a popular slogan then.

Jane Fonda's fitness techniques and aerobic workout changed my entire body. I loved the way it felt and what it did for me. I had been a kid who could never touch my toes. I'd never worked out, wasn't athletic, and had started to gain weight. A friend turned me on to all this exercising. She was studying nutrition at Tufts University while working at a Jack LaLanne health club (which were the only fitness studios around at the time). I fell in love with working out, because it helped me feel great, besides giving my physique an entire makeover.

Following the Trends

During my early career days, gyms and studios were just beginning to open, and the classes that were available were mostly high impact. You also could find studios that taught dancing classes, but that was really it. The trend then shifted to low impact as people started getting hurt. Then step fitness and slide classes became in vogue—and then went right out again!

Yoga and Pilates were always available; yoga has been widely offered in the West since the 1960s. But these two forms of exercise were thought of as elite forms of fitness back in the day. People started to practice yoga and Pilates in earnest only as they became injured from the trendy high-impact classes.

In recent years we've seen other types of low impact trends, from Zumba to Doonya, Drums Alive and Nia, even Belly dance has shown up on the fitness circuits and there are so many different variations on the Bar class. These are fun and social ways of varying your routine. .

There is no shortage of classes featuring the latest trends for physical workouts, like spin cycling and hard-core boot camps but the most positive trend comes in the form of nutrition. The *Am New York* website (amNY.com) says New York is "the hottest vegan city," which is another trend. As fitness becomes part of the forefront activity in people's lives, they naturally seek healthier food. And there is no shortage of it here.

Currently, high-intensity fitness training is all the rage. During these classes you'll experience short spurts of high intensity followed by a short period of rest and recovery. Barry's Boot camp and any other studio that offers Cross Fit training classes are great examples of this trend. However, I believe the Cross Fit trend will probably evolve because while the challenge is exhilarating people are getting hurt if they go into these classes without proper guidance.

Commercialization and branding are where I see the fitness trends heading in the near future. There are a lot of classes with gimmicks funded by venture capital, and those studios are looking for the masses to participate. I see the burst of spinning classes as one type of trend that has gained a lot of traction. Each studio is trying to outdo the other with specialty, and most of these studios are consistently crowded. They're modern, competitive, hip, and young. The music is loud in most of the places (so much so that some studios even offer earplugs at their front desks!). I've even seen some places adding spinning yoga to their mixes and being more and more creative with their class offerings. Spinning is not dying out anytime soon, but it's not for everyone. You either love it or you hate it, but you most definitely get a workout.

The health and wellness craze is attracting serious investments into branding their approach, elevating the industry to a new level of hype, especially in New York. The current trend among the hottest studios is for bigger, better equipment. The studios are beautiful and make you feel good, and the people who own and manage them are community minded. Examples of this type of studio are SoulCycle, New York Pilates, Core Pilates, SLT (short for Strengthen, Lengthen, Tone), and Flywheel Sports. Their goal is to create a brand in addition to an exercise studio. Many of them offer clothing lines featuring their names. They seek to become communities as well as commercialized products.

The Trend for More Instructor Education

At the beginning of my career, nobody was certified. Very little formal training was available. Teaching was just a matter of looking good and having a passion for fitness, plus being able to get up in front of a group and control the crowd. That's how you got the job as an instructor. People just liked to work out, and class instruction was very superficial.

At the time, people were starting to enjoy the trend of being in classes with others. They liked the energy they got from it. They didn't necessarily like the pain of working out, but they discovered the wonderful way they felt physically afterward. Fitness back then was about being in a group, together, sweating. It was about endorphins. And it was about seeing changes in the body and feeling good.

I was one of the lucky ones; a company that did corporate fitness formally trained me in the Pilates mat style of working out. Then in 1985 a certification was offered in what is called group fitness for the first time, and I was in one of the first groups of certified teachers.

But even then I didn't know about the human body the way I know it now. And at that time, I thought Pilates was so strange, because everyone started out on the floor to do their workouts. I didn't know it was Pilates. I incorporated Jane Fonda's techniques with the Pilates work done on the mat (a combination workout). And because Jane Fonda was the trend of the day, I relied more on her style of teaching in the beginning of my career than I did Pilates.

I trained a former Miss Universe, Yvonne Ryding, at Club La Raquette at the Le Parker Meridian Hotel. We designed a fitness video together in 1987. From 1983 to 1986, I also designed the morning workout at Club La Raquette for corporate fitness clients as well as other high-profile clients before opening Irene's Fitness Studio in 1986, where I launched my own unique style of training programs.

After that the industry changed, because people craved knowing more about fitness, their bodies, and their health. As that desire increased, more education for instructors became available. Today's trend is that instructors want to know more, and online education is available to them. The fitness training industry is expected to grow by 23 percent in the next ten years, according to the US Bureau of Labor Statistics, so it's crucial for trainers to be educated. Instructors can do so much more research so much more easily. New certification programs are popping up every day, and everybody wants to have a certifying teaching studio. And let's face it—there's a lot of money in that!

You can find any type of course, and the number of courses is overwhelming! For example, almost every year I do a functional anatomy class at Mount Sinai Hospital. I study cadavers to learn about the body, which is important because I'm working with my clients' bodies. It's fascinating seeing the body parts and what I'm actually doing when I'm helping someone to exercise. To see all the organs, muscles, and the bones; to hold someone's brain in my hands—it really does help with my teaching. I can see these organs and muscles in my mind's eye, and when someone tells me what's going on physically with them, I can visualize internally what that person is experiencing.

The more you know, the more you can do for a person. This is the type of thing that is available to instructors now.

The Trend of Reinvention

Classic and contemporary Pilates classes are still prominent because of their long-term results. More and more studios are incorporating Pilates in their ideology, which continues to reinvent the practice as an addition like "flex" Pilates (which combines traditional Pilates and dynamic strength training) and Chair Pilates have all received acclaim. Similarly, chaise fitness is a new spin on chair Pilates. Joseph Pilates originally created the chair used in chair Pilates as a home exercise machine, and the early design converted from a chair to sit on to a chair to exercise with, known as the Wunda chair. It is a simple piece of equipment—a seat, a pedal, and springs that attach to the pedal to create resistance.

Yoga also remains popular. Yoga has been around for five thousand years and gained popularity during the twentieth century. The hype surrounding it has exploded exponentially in recent years. Yoga is everywhere, from the popular hot yoga to Vinyasa flow to restorative and slow flow. One reinvention of this five-thousand-year-old practice is Antigravity aerial yoga, in which a hammock acts as a soft trapeze and supports you while you work on simple inversions and progress to those that are more advanced.

There is a yoga practice and studio for everyone. However, yoga isn't everyone's preferred method of finding fitness. I much prefer hanging from a Pilates Cadillac (which is a specialized piece of Pilates equipment that tones every muscle group) to doing headstands and handstands. But I still love the flow of the sun salutation and the floor work of various Yoga Asana, which stretch me and make my body feel good. And who doesn't love Savasana (corpse pose)? If yoga is your thing, you will always find benefits by incorporating it into your life, and you'll always find plentiful studio options.

Yoga means "union," and that's quite apropos for fitness seekers. It's about the union of the body, mind, and spirit. It brings people together. Maybe you're not a naturally flexible person. That can discourage some people from even trying yoga, but keep in mind that yoga is a practice, and you will become more flexible over time. The wonder of yoga is you can go at your own pace. It's not about pushing; it's about easing into each position with no pain and no judgment.

Another trend that has been reinvented is semiprivate personal training, in which two or three people meet with a trainer at an appointed time.

Then you have your high-end clients looking for personalization and one-on-one attention as they work on their preferred methods of exercise.

*As a special note: Flexibility and joint limitations should be considered when experiencing different forms of exercise. Our flexibility can be endless with consistency and can improve but should never be forced. Your body is different from others. Your physical, genetic disposition should not be compared to another or manipulated into doing something it wasn't meant to do because your personal anatomy can affect your range of motion.

Hot New Trend

A hot new trend gaining momentum is fitness classes through online streaming. It seems you can get any kind of workout or fitness information you crave on line and set up so you can follow along. Some studios now allow you join their classes from home.

Fitness for Young and Old

The obesity epidemic in this country is unbelievable, and I don't see that getting better anytime soon. One-third of the population in the United States is clinically obese, and one billion people worldwide are over their ideal weight.

One particular group fighting this problem is children. As a result, exercise programs geared specifically for children are becoming more and more popular at fitness studios. Certifications are now being offered for children's fitness programs. So it is important to look for well-qualified professionals. Some of the children's fitness trends include sports-specific training, Cross Fit, yoga, Zumba, and even personal training, to name a few.

There are efforts beginning now to offer at schools a Pilates style fitness program to help teach children how to stand, sit and breathe properly. Re-evaluating students chairs and providing stools as well as a ball chairs will help admonish the daily damage to children's posture.

Exercise programs specifically geared toward older adults are more available as baby boomers are staying in better shape, so it is in the interest of fitness studios to tailor classes for them for years to come. Studios are making sure they offer lower-impact workout alternatives and are incorporating "functional fitness" into workouts for senior adults which is aiding in the activities they would do in everyday normal life, like carrying grocery bags and standing and sitting.

Balance training should also be a key component in a senior adult fitness routine. My personal recommendation for seniors is to practice balance every day. Any qualified senior instructor will make sure that you will find a focus on balance.

The Unexpected Pain from the Trends

The benefit of trendy studios is that you can jump into a class almost anytime. Most offer classes every hour, so if you have a busy schedule, you'll have no problem finding a workout.

With that said, you need to have a balance. To find that balance, you have to really listen to your body. With a mass market and trendy fitness studio, you may go to a class and afterward feel like it gave you the hard workout you needed. But what did you really accomplish during that class? People who seek the "no pain, no gain" type of workout, almost feel like they were beaten up; and isn't that what a workout should feel like? Does being in pain mean progress? Not always. Sometimes pain means you actually end up with an injury.

Doing something different all the time helps you get great cross training, but at the end of the day, it doesn't always mean maximum muscle gain or weight management. You're just piling on new movements that your body isn't used to doing. So you may ask what is the solution? It is better to build consistency in a workout regimen. By building consistency, you begin to know what you are doing, and if know what you are doing, you won't get hurt and then you will receive fitness goals. As long as you're moving and feeling good during the movements, there are benefits to almost anything. Your body is meant to move. It feels good to move.

We are not meant to sit in chairs all day. There are even many options for treadmill desks so that you can walk while you work and I see this as a trend of the future. They say sitting is like the new smoking and we know how bad that is for your body. Plus you can burn three to five times more calories while you work.

It all comes back to listening to your body and doing what feels good and safe. You don't have to kill yourself. The second you feel something is not right, ease up or stop doing the exercise. Just because everyone else is doing it in your class doesn't mean it's right for your body.

For example, if I go to a boot camp class and am told to run up a hill at ten miles per hour, I'll go at my own pace, because that's good for my body. As you get older, I believe, you still need to work hard but at a different level—not jumping up and down and killing it. After a while your body's going to rebel. We're delicate. We really are! We can abuse our bodies in trying to be super fit.

If you are pursuing hard-core classes right now, doing them every day is not going to do your body justice. If you love a hard-core workout and are young and/or able to do it, it's fine as long, as you're intelligently cautious and don't do the workouts too much in a given week. If you feel the need to "beat yourself up" physically from time to time, that's fine, but stay away from the repetitive practice, unless you are a professional athlete under supervision..

You should balance hard-core workouts with taking fitness walks. (I love my pedometer, which tells me how many steps I walk in a day—anything to encourage more movement.) If you are sitting at a desk all day, do something in the chair that moves your body. On the day when you don't go to class, walk everywhere, or take a yoga or Pilates class. Add in a hard-core class once or twice a week at most. Always be naturally moving.

In addition, take a few minutes every day just to breathe and focus on your breath. Fill your lungs with air. Just thinking about that will help you move better and more frequently.

The bottom line is this: you work out because it feels good, it makes you look good, and so you see long-term benefits, one of which is helping you to move for the rest of your life.

If you abuse your body, you'll lose that last thing. You want to be able to easily get out of bed and on and off the floor when you're eighty years old. You want to move freely. I see people who looked great in their thirties and early forties, but by the time they turned fifty, they could hardly move because they have had so many injuries. They have abused their bodies with heavy weights and Cross Fit training, but the long-term benefits weren't there. Today they're moving like old people instead of vibrant fifty-year-olds.

You want to find things you like and that are fun for you and keep you moving but also that keep you moving safely.

If you feel accomplished and high after your workout, then your workout is great. If you feel like crap and you can't move, it doesn't mean you're closer to making changes in your body. The key to working out and taking classes is that you want to do it for the rest of your life, and you want to be able to move freely for the rest of your life.

As long as you listen to your body during your workouts, even challenging fitness trends can be wonderful additions to your quest to find balance and fitness.

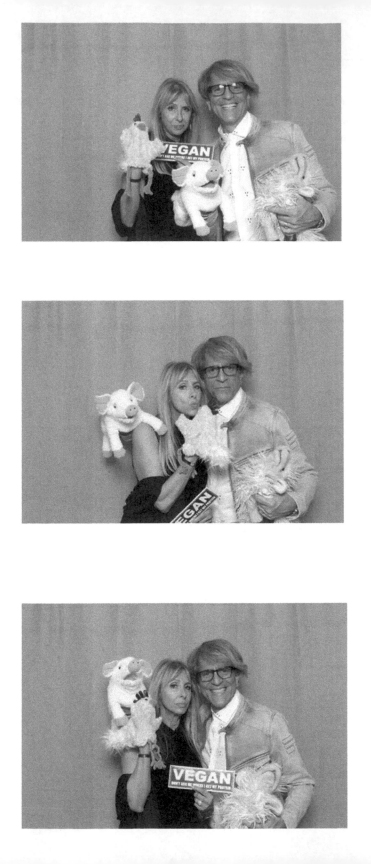

Finding Beauty and Joy

When you seek beauty in all people and all things,
you will not only find it, you will become it.
—ANONYMOUS

Just like the good witch in *The Wizard of Oz* told Dorothy, "It's been there all along. Joy is within in you and is enhanced by external things."

Most people do not place enough awareness on what makes them happy. Consumed with everyday life and being "busy," often we forget to create the moments that bring us joy.

So let me ask you to think about this question: How do you find the joy within you?

I find joy in exercise, plant-based foods, and being with my family and friends. I find joy in making someone else happy. Movement brings me joy. Knowing I do something for my body and soul every day adds joy too. I place high importance on creating fun in my life. I do believe it's important to make myself look and feel good.

Let's discover some ways to inject health, energy, joy, and beauty into your life.

Fit Fun

Nobody dies from feeling good!

Make sure that every once in a while, you find a reason to celebrate. Enjoy anything that's a celebration of life. Do random acts of kindness. Be conscious of what you're eating; savor food. Take time to do and think about things you enjoy doing and thinking about. Have a night out.

Most of the dates I have with my husband, my daughter, my son, and even my sister and sometimes my parents involve fit nights, days, and weekends. Instead of going out for dinner and drinks, for example, plan your activity so that you do a fitness class together from 6:00 to 8:00 p.m., and then head out for a nice meal and an invigorating walk around your town or city. Living in New York, I have a vast array of choices, and I like to indulge in them all.

When people hear I walk from Thirtieth Street to SoHo, they're amazed. But each and every neighborhood is a hidden gem. Besides getting great exercise, I discover the beauty and joy of these community jewels. Almost every area is much more upscale now than it was in the past, and beauty is everywhere I look. Most areas are really interesting, with cool shops and great clothing stores. Every area has something in it that's enjoyable—for example, its own vegan restaurants and exercise classes, not to mention movie theaters, shows, and museums. There is no area in New York where you can't find something you need or want.

I use a bracelet pedometer to keep track of how many steps I'm taking. I find it's nothing for me to take fifteen thousand steps. That's the beauty of it. I'm walking, exploring, and seeing. There are beautiful places to go everywhere. In any city or suburb, I can find many hidden treasures, and so can you.

Besides walking, we have several ice-skating rinks in New York City. There's always something you can do for fit fun, and it doesn't have to be a class at a studio. And if you just find joy in watching the skaters or going to Radio City Music Hall, those are amazing experiences in and of itself. My family and I go to on and off Broadway shows regularly. We also go to museums once in a while and seek out new music venues. You should never be lacking for things to do.. Discovery is a wonderful tool for fitness.

Everything is available in this city as I am sure in most cities across the USA, but it's up to you to find what you think is fun; also make sure you take time for the things you enjoy wherever you live. And during a night out, find joy in the things that benefit you, like good food, but even comfort food can be healthier and compassionate.. We have very powerful minds, and our minds and bodies are connected. We can choose to eat well and do good things for our bodies, or we can ignore the things we need. Don't get off track and hit a place that offers food that I call "a heart attack on a plate." Sure, the line may be out the door and down the sidewalk, but is that food really worth it? When you start adopting the good habit of indulging in activities and food that make you feel joyful and not deprived, you are doing something good for your body and taking on a new mind-set at the same time.

Indulge in a Beautiful You

Anything that pampers you and makes you feel good is a good thing. As long as we're here on this planet, we might as well take care of ourselves! Enjoy taking care of yourself!

Facials are great. I never regularly indulged in facials until a client once gave me a gift certificate for one, and then I discovered how wonderful they are. Getting facials as well as massages are both things you should do, and there are plenty of spas around most cities and towns. There are also a lot of late night manicure and pedicure spots in New York.

Good poops are a big health conversation for me with my clients. Ideally you should poop more than once a day. You eat more than once a day, so your body should eliminate waste regularly to feel healthy and look radiantly glowing.

I think part of beauty and joy is proper nutrition. When you eat right, you feel so much better, and your skin looks so much better. Eat a lot of greens. Make sure you have breakfast. One of the worst mistakes people make is not eating breakfast. And chew your food well. The more you chew, the less work your body has to do.

I am also a big fan of detoxing at least once a year, like at the We Care Detox Spa and Spiritual Retreat. It's important to detox. The skin is the largest organ of elimination. Detoxing baths are great for you too. And let's face it—it's a luxury to take the time to take a bath! It's a relaxing treat, and it's a nice thing to do for you.

My tip to clear away toxins daily is threefold: breathing, dry brushing, and hydration.

1. Breathing is so important. Most people don't take full breaths and breathe into their lungs; they don't fill their lungs with air and get their ribs moving. My philosophy is that the post lateral breath (breathing deep into the back and the rib cage) is highly important. As we get older, breathing becomes even more important to our upper thoracic area. We need full breaths in the lungs, because our ribs are meant to move.

    Belly breathing is one element I see practiced in yoga, which is a wonderful practice for when you are doing yoga and also if you are taking voice lessons, as long as you are also regularly practicing post lateral breathing. Please keep those ribs moving, those lungs filling with air. Remember, the breath is meant to fill the lungs and keep those ribs from getting stiff. I encourage people to adopt Dr. Andrew Weil's breathing technique: inhale for four counts, hold your breath for seven counts, exhale for eight counts, and then repeat the sequence four times. It releases tension in the body. When someone who is tense comes into my studio, I have him or her do that breathing exercise, so that by the end of the session, he or she is breathing properly again.

2. Dry brushing opens the pores and is good for you. It stimulates your skin, and you'll look and feel better. Use a dry brush to get rid of dead layers of skin. It's a regular practice for me before I get into the shower.

3. Hydration is good for your skin and weight loss, so drink up. Take your body weight, and divide it by two. That number is the total ounces of water you should be drinking daily. That said, you might be surprised to learn that I recommend against drinking with your meals. It dilutes the digestive juices that break down the food. Drink half an hour before your meals and two hours after your meals. For most people this would be difficult, but as soon as I wake, I consume one twenty-ounce bottle of water. I drink an additional twenty ounces with my vitamins; and I take another twenty ounces of water as I travel to work. So before my day begins, I have already consumed my daily allowance for hydration, and anything after that is a bonus for a fitter, healthier body.

Sinking into Meditation and Joy

Meditation is so important. It forces you to take the time out you need to cleanse your mind, stress less, and sink into the joy of living. It reminds you to live consciously. It helps you to nurture yourself. It takes just ten minutes a day to offer your body a personal meditation, and the benefits you reap will be astounding.

Make sure your home surroundings are comforting. Scents play a huge role in feeling the beauty and feeling joyful, plus they give you the power to breathe better. In my shower I spray eucalyptus every day, so I feel like I'm in a spa. It also opens the lungs and clears the nasal passages. Every morning in my studio, I spray peppermint, which is good to enhance energy; it also alleviates headaches and nausea. Essential oils do help. They stimulate your senses. I'm a big believer in them. I also regularly use lavender, because it's relaxing. For a list of essential oils and their benefits, go to www.mydoterra.com/daraekster.

And let's not forget about music. You can use music as a way of creating moods and expressing movement through dancing. I use music in my studio, because it does create a feeling and a sensation. Sometimes, if you just let go, listen, dance, and enjoy the music, it's a good thing for your state of mind. When cooking dinner, putting on music and dancing adds movement to what you're doing, so you're not just standing at a stove. Our bodies are meant to move. The more you can enjoy movement, the more you will enjoy life.

So many people believe that alcohol is the key to a fun social life. But in reality alcohol dehydrates, so if you are going to indulge, it's best to make sure you also drink at least one glass of water for every portion of alcohol you consume. Also, you can make healthier choices and enjoy an organic, vegan wine or liquor. An informative list can be found at barnivore.com.

Sleep and Streamlined Living

When you feel and do things that are healthy for you, you'll be thinking positively in no time.

Sleep is undervalued in our society. So sleep deeply. Get your seven hours of recommended shut-eye. Cut off all lights and blacken the room if possible. A healthy choice to help you sleep is Natural Calm, which is a magnesium supplement. Go to naturalvitality.com for more information.

We walk around in a chronic state of stress. Address stress before you hit the pillow. Use relaxation techniques so you can handle difficult discussions. There are many relaxation audios and apps available; one I always recommend is Deepak Chopra's 21-Day Meditation, or search to see which ones suit you best. Remember, it takes only five to ten minutes a day to bring you back to a relaxed state of mind.

Surround yourself with beauty. Organize your home. Bring home fresh flowers. Your refrigerator and cabinets should be organized so that there is streamlined thinking. This also simplifies and de-stresses your life. People don't realize the power of an organized refrigerator on their frame of mind when it comes to eating food that's good for them. Take a lovely photo of something from nature and put it on the refrigerator so that it becomes another welcoming place.

Adore solutions.

Breathe deeply.

Love more.

Live the good life.

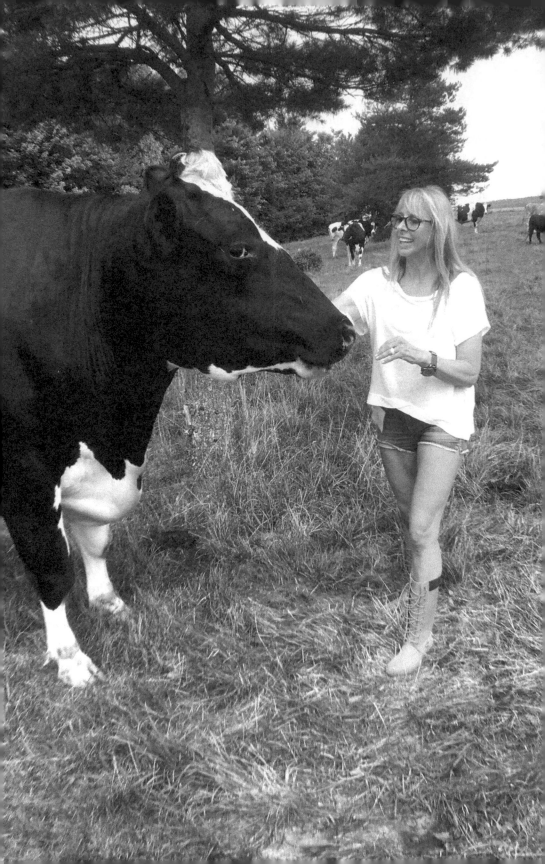

Finding Compassion

Nothing will benefit human health and increase
the chances for survival of life on earth as much
as the evolution to a vegetarian diet.
—ALBERT EINSTEIN

The vegan diet is the highest praise a
human can give to life on earth.
—IRENE RIZZO

When I look into the eyes of an animal, I do not see an
animal I see a living being. I see a friend. I feel a soul.
—A. D. WILLIAMS

There is no fundamental difference between man and animals
in their ability to feel pleasure and pain, happiness, and misery.
—CHARLES DARWIN

The new mother's labor had finally come to an end. The agonizing birthing pain was already a memory. Joy filled her heart as her newborn's cries reached her ears. She was exhausted, but she was thrilled. At long last her baby was here, and she couldn't wait to see him.

She looked to the attending midwife expectantly, waiting for the baby to be brought to her. Already she could feel her breasts tingle as milk filled them, and she prepared herself to provide her infant with his first nourishment of his life.

Then it happened—the real-life nightmare she never saw coming.

Rather than bringing the baby to her, the midwife turned her back to the mother and, cradling him in her arms, walked right out of the room with him.

The baby screamed.

"Where are you going with my baby?" the mother wailed.

Milk was now soaking her skin as the sound of the baby's cries automatically triggered her body into producing more of it. She could hear the baby in another room, continuing to cry for her.

"What is happening to my baby? Where is my baby?" the mother cried, now frantic.

No one answered. It was as if she was invisible.

She started screaming. "Where is he? Bring him to me this instant! I want my baby! I want my baby!"

What happened next was any mother's worst fear. Through a window in the room, she could see people handling her baby. What were they doing to him? They were putting him in a wooden box! He continued to cry as the people took the box outside of the building. She heard the sound of a truck and the *thump-thump* of the box being tossed into its bed. The baby's faint cries disappeared as the truck drove away.

The mother cried, moaned, wailed, and sobbed.

"Where did you take my baby? Where is my baby? What have you done with him?"

But no one would answer her. In fact no one could understand her wordless pleading...for her protests were not uttered in human language.

The mother was a dairy cow.

This is a scene that happens repeatedly in dairy barns, as calves are taken from their mothers within minutes of being born. The males go to veal farms. The females are separated for their future fate as milk producers.

And all the while, the mothers can hear the babies crying for them, which triggers their bodies into making more milk—and, ultimately, more money for the dairy farmer.

You may think, well, these are just animals, a piece of inventory for a food business. What does it matter? But you would be wrong. Cows are very intelligent and can remember things for a long time. They interact in socially complex ways. They also are known to mourn the deaths of and separations from other animals, even shedding tears.

Perhaps one of the most profound testimonies about the emotions of cows comes from Michael Klaper, MD, who is regarded as the voice of the vegan movement and is an American physician who practices preventative and nutrition-based medicine. He is director of the Institute of Nutrition Education and Research and has served as a nutritional advisor to NASA.

Dr. Klaper spent sixteen childhood summers on his uncle's Wisconsin dairy farm, which is where he had his own unique encounter with cows and their terrible fates:

> The very saddest sound in all my memory was burned into my awareness at age five on my uncle's dairy farm in Wisconsin. A cow had given birth to a beautiful male calf. The mother was allowed to nurse her calf but for a single night. On the second day after birth, my uncle took the calf from the mother and placed him in the veal pen in the barn—only ten yards away, in plain view of the mother. The mother cow could see her infant, smell him, hear him, but could not touch him, comfort him, or nurse him. The heartrending bellows that she poured forth—minute after minute, hour after hour, for five long days—were excruciating to listen to. They are the most poignant and painful auditory memories I carry in my brain.
>
> Since that age, whenever I hear anyone postulate that animals cannot feel emotions, I need only to replay that torturous sound in my memory of that mother cow crying her bovine heart out to her infant. Mother's love knows no species barriers, and I believe that all people who are vegans in their hearts and souls know that to be true.[1]

I'd like to walk you through a dairy barn to show you what happens.

You'll see the mother cows hooked up to machines several times a day. You may see artificial insemination taking place, to keep cows continually pregnant, so they keep making the milk for your cereal.

According to People for the Ethical Treatment of Animals (PETA), the cows are often drugged "to force them to produce about four-and-a-half times as much milk as they naturally would to feed their calves."[2]

If you've ever nursed a baby, you're probably familiar with mastitis, a painful inflammation of the mammary glands. The dairy industry reports that 30–50 percent of

---

1 Michael Klaper, "Vegan: A Dairy Cow Story with a Happy Ending," December 9, 2011. www.gluten-freeveganmom.com.

2 PETA, "The Dairy Industry: Cows Used for Milk," www.peta.org.

dairy cows suffer from it. What contributes to it is the bovine growth hormone (BGH), with which the cows are dosed.

Oh, and let's not forget about the life span. As you gaze around this dairy barn, be aware that the cows you are seeing will live for an average of four to five years. And if they don't die of natural causes, the dairy industry kills them, because by the time they reach that age, nearly 40 percent are lame "because of the intensive confinement, the filth and the strain of being almost always pregnant and giving milk," says PETA.[3] What's the average age of a cow that does not live under these conditions? Twenty-five years!

Gary Yourofsky is an animal-rights activist who has spoken to thousands of students about animal rights. In one such speech, which is captured on YouTube, Yourofsky noted that 90 percent of hamburger meat in America comes from the dairy industry.

"When cows no longer give huge amounts of milk after three to seven years—slaughterhouse, no exceptions," he says.[4]

The whole scenario for one dairy cow is simply horrifying and torturous. An animal suffers so you can enjoy a cold glass of milk or butter on your bread—a taste you don't have to give up and can easily achieve with cashew and almond butters and products like Earth Balance. As for milk alternatives, there is a wide variety: soy, almond, hemp, oat, coconut, rice, almond/coconut, and quinoa. There is at least one vegan alternative for everyone's taste.

And if this is what goes on in a dairy barn, the slaughterhouses have their own brand of torture for the animals that are slaughtered for our daily consumption. Paul McCartney, who is a vegetarian, once said, "If a slaughterhouse had glass walls, everyone would be a vegetarian."

Even the transport to the slaughterhouse can be torturous. On its website, MercyforAnimals.ca, Mercy for Animals in Canada provides disturbing undercover footage of horrific animal cruelty in Alberta, Canada. The site says,

> This case graphically illustrates the cruel and inhumane treatment that farmed animals are all too often subjected to during transport. Canada's outdated livestock transport regulations are downright shameful, and lag behind the rest of the Western world. As a result, pigs and other farmed animals are often

---

3   Ibid.
4   Gary Yourofsky, "The Best Speech You Will Ever Hear," YouTube, http://youtu.be/es6U00LMmC4.

trucked thousands of kilometers for up to 52 hours at a time without any food, water, or rest, resulting in the deaths of over eight million animals a year.

Just taking our dairy barn as one example, you can see that the treatment of these animals is heartless. For us, as the higher species, it's in our nature to want to do something about it.

That's where a plant-based diet is vital.

Vegetarianism begins in your heart. It begins with the understanding of what life really is and where your food comes from. It reaches beyond even your own personal health concerns.

It's about finding compassion.

That's why a plant-based lifestyle is very important to me. If I look at a chicken sandwich for lunch, I don't see it just as food or something maybe unhealthy, I also think, a being probably suffered in order for me to have this.

My belief is that if we interviewed every human being on the planet, all would consider themselves compassionate. But if you tell people about the plight of an animal like a dairy cow, they will turn away. Why is it that we ignore these very clear cases of cruelty? It's because people still want to be able to eat dairy and meat—and the root of that desire is an addiction to habits, lack of knowledge, and lack of resources to practice healthier and tastier non-animal-product alternatives.

When you ingest meat, you're not doing your body any favors. In his YouTube speech, Yourofsky noted,

> The length of our intestines are somewhere between seven to thirteen times the length of our torso, our trunk. That's the same length of all herbivore animal intestines on this planet. They're very long. But the length of the intestines on real meat eaters, hyenas, coyotes, bears, tigers and lions, only three to six times the length of their torso. They have a short intestinal tract, so they can push through quickly, decaying and rotting animal flesh.[5]

As Yourofsky eloquently pointed out, the theory that humans are natural carnivores is just not true. Watch Yourofsky's compelling and convincing speech, which he gave on March 24, 2014, at City College–New York.

---

5 Yourofsky, "Best Speech."

Melanie Joy, PhD, Ed.M., is a Harvard-educated psychologist; professor of psychology and sociology at the University of Massachusetts, Boston; and author of the award winning book *Why We Love Dogs, Eat Pigs, and Wear Cows*. She coined the word *Carnism*, which she defines as "the invisible belief system that shapes our perceptions of the meat we eat, so that we love some animals and eat others without knowing why."[6]

She brings up a great point in her book about the meat industry: "As with any violent ideology, the populace must be shielded from direct exposure to the victims of the system, lest they begin questioning the system or their participation in it. This truth speaks for itself: why else would the meat industry go to such lengths to keep its practices invisible?"[7]

Those are my feelings exactly, and that's the foundation for my view that if you want to find compassion, you must look at the entirety of the world around you—not just things that affect your quality of life but also things that affect the lives of all living creatures. That compassion, in turn, feeds into your overall quality of life.

For example, I know that a diet rich in fruit, vegetables, and grains—which have equal amounts of protein to meat—doesn't affect just my physical heart health. It also strengthens my emotional heart. I know my choice not to eat meat creates less of a demand for the suffering of other creatures.

How I Found Compassion—and, Later, Health

My strong focus on health and fitness has been with me since I was very young. And it all started because of my older brother, Jeff, and a conversation at the dinner table when I was eleven years old.

Jeff was a student at MIT, and he'd just come home for a visit. We sat down as a family for dinner, and he asked me a question that stopped my fork in midair.

"Do you realize you're eating a chicken?"

He knew how much I loved animals. All of a sudden, it clicked. What I had on my plate was an actual animal. It never would have occurred to me until then that this was the case. From that moment on, I could never eat meat again. I'm not sure if my brother expected me to stop eating meat for the rest of my life, but that was the effect of his one sentence.

---

6 "Why We Love Dogs, Eat Pigs, and Wear Cows," CAAN, Awareness and Action Network, www.carnism.org.

7 Ibid.

Intuition told me eating animals was wrong. I had become aware of what my food actually was. But even at that point, I did not associate abuse with animal-based diets. At the time, it was enough for me to know that an animal had to die for me to eat. As I got older, however, I learned more about disturbing practices, like what dairy cows experience when giving milk. As my compassion for their plight deepened, I also became more fully immersed in the health benefits of a 100 percent plant-based lifestyle on the human body and the emotional psyche.

Besides slaughtering animals for their meat, we kill them to fulfill other "needs." This is another thing I learned, as I got older. I never realized, for example, that the shoes I wore and the fabrics I put on my body were from animals. There are plenty that are tortured for their fur. I learned about a lot of disturbing practices, including how the cosmetic industry harms animals for testing.

It all came together for me. Each part of the total picture was connected to another, and when the picture was complete, it was all about healthy and compassionate living. I realized that there is not much difference between eating your dog and eating your pig. Melanie Joy eloquently gives the example of a dinner party at which people are complimenting the hostess on the delicious meat course, only to discover they are eating a golden retriever. Her point with this made-up scenario is that people will often consume ham or steaks without realizing the animals they're eating had personalities and feelings, much like dogs do. They would never consider eating a pet dog, but they have no problem taking part in the eating of a cow or pig, an animal that would respond to human kindness in the same manner as a dog would.

You may remember the "Mad Cowboy," Howard Lyman, and his appearance on the *Oprah Show*. He told the truth about the beef industry, and Oprah said she'd never eat meat again. They were sued by Texas cattlemen for slander, but in 2002 the lawsuit was dismissed without prejudice.

The meat and dairy industries are so powerful that we are still being told dairy is good for us. Dr. Walter Willett, chair of Harvard University's Department of Nutrition, says the hype surrounding milk and the dairy industry is misleading—and he even comes from a long line of dairy farmers! People believe that consuming a lot of milk will prevent osteoporosis and fractures. But Dr. Willett says, "Studies that have looked at milk and dairy consumption do not show that people who drink more cow's milk have lower fracture risk."[8]

---

8 Sharon Kirkey, "Drinking Milk Not Essential for Humans Despite Belief It Prevents Osteoporosis, Nutritionist Says," Postmedia News, http://life.nationalpost.com/2014/01/23/drinking-milk-not-essential-for-humans-despite-belief-it-prevents-osteoporosis-nutritionist-says/.

In January 2014 Willett and his colleagues published research in the *JAMA Pediatrics* journal on ninety-six thousand people who had participated in two-decades-long studies. The results showed that "high milk consumption during the teen years didn't translate into a lower risk of hip fractures when people got older."[9]

For me, a plant-based diet is not just about health, however. Yes, I am a health coach and I do help people to get healthier, lose weight, and feel better. My decision goes beyond that. It's also about being compassionate to other living creatures.

When I started with a plant-based lifestyle, not a lot of people were doing what I was doing. But it affected my heart, and it was in my heart.

It was who I am.

Compassionate Choices Equal Better Living

Today I tell my clients that everything I do is connected to something I feel. When you receive this understanding—when you become passionate about realizing things other people don't see—it's a true gift. It makes life all the more worth living as you give back to the world around you with your compassionate choices. Not only that, but compassionate living leads to a healthier and longer life.

This isn't as complicated as you think it may be. If you are eating healthily, you never have to think about dieting. You never have to think about high cholesterol.

Here's your personal challenge: Take a blood test, and get your cholesterol reading and your performance measurements for your kidneys and liver, plus your levels of vitamin D and vitamin C. Then switch over to a plant-based diet for a period of one year. In twelve months, follow up with another test. You will be astonished by the results. I predict you'll have a lot more energy and vibrancy than you ever did before. You also will probably experience fewer colds and viruses, especially if they are a routine occurrence for you currently. Not only that, but you'll love the way you look! You'll lose weight and see a lean physique when you look in the mirror. Your skin will become more vibrant and fresh.

Hippocrates, the father of Western medicine, said, "Let food be thy medicine and medicine be thy food." I'm a strong believer in those words. I believe in the power of food to lead you to finding great health. I believe eating the right way and changing what you put into your mouth can actually lead you to finding the Mountain of Youth.

Think about this: the only foods with cholesterol are animal products.

---

9 Ibid.

Eliminate meat, dairy, and eggs, and you will see a shift in how you look and feel—and in your health. All of the protein you need, all of the calcium and vitamins you need, are in plants and whole grains.

Dr. Neal D. Barnard is a clinical researcher, an author, and one of America's leading advocates for health, nutrition, and higher standards in research. He is also the principal investigator of several human clinical research trials, the results of which are published in peer-reviewed medical and scientific journals. His book is called *Dr. Neal Barnard's Program for Reversing Diabetes* (2007, Rodale). He has also written *Power Foods for the Brain, 21-Day Weightloss Kickstart, The Get Healthy, Go Vegan Cookbook,* and *Breaking the Food Seduction.*

Dr. Barnard points to studies that show that by adopting a low-fat vegetarian diet (free of all animal products and added vegetable oils), you can lower your cholesterol, reduce your blood pressure, and lose weight. And you can reverse diabetes. Dr. Barnard's program helps repair how the body uses insulin.

Dr. Joel Fuhrman is another medical doctor who can similarly attest to this lifestyle. He is the author of *Eat to Live* and counsels patients on his "nutritarian" lifestyle. In coining this phrase, he tries to bring an understanding that a nutritarian lifestyle has a powerful disease-preventing and therapeutic effect on the body. So it is important to consume a broad array of micronutrients via their food choices. Foods that are highest in micronutrients are green leafy and colorful vegetables; fruits such cherries, berries, and oranges. He is also an athlete who advises athletes on proper nutrition for optimal performance.

Yet even with the strong backing of members of the medical community, you still may be skeptical that a plant-based diet is right for you. And there's one myth that is probably standing in your way from fully embracing it.

Proteins

Protein is the number-one concern I hear from people who are cautious about moving to a vegan or vegetarian diet. If you think you can get your protein only from meat, that's societal brainwashing. You can get all the protein you need through beans, which also have fiber. The best sources of protein are garbanzo beans and kidney beans as well as peanut butter, tofu,, almonds, and cashews. In addition, every vegetable has some amount of protein in it. Broccoli derives 49 percent of its calories from protein.

Most Americans eat way more protein than they need. And many meat eaters don't know that getting excess protein can cause health problems, like kidney stones and some cancers. A diet based on beans and vegetables provides an adequate amount without the risk of protein overdose.

I don't worry about my protein as a vegan. As long as I'm eating a plate of vegetables, I'm getting it. You also don't have to worry about getting enough protein. If you still are concerned, I suggest using Sun Warrior Protein Powder in smoothies. And a rice protein is excellent. Beans are one of my favorite sources. You get protein from everything you eat—all vegetables have some in it.

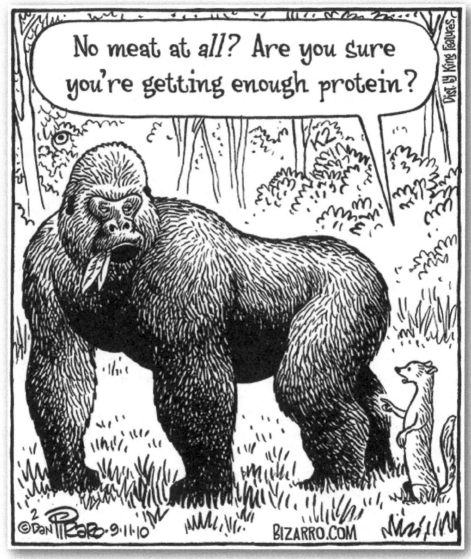

"Reprinted by permission of Dan Piraro"

Vegan and Vegetarian Athletes and Celebrities

Let's look at athletes and celebrities as an example of why you can get by without meat protein. Many athletes are told from a young age to eat protein, they translate *protein* as chicken, beef, and fish. I have seen many clients feed their athletic children meat for breakfast, lunch, and dinner. And I've seen many children get sick. Did you know that meat protein is much more difficult to digest than plant-based proteins? Your body has to work harder to break down the amino acids in meat and slows down your digestion and often will make you feel sluggish. In comparison, plant proteins will digest relatively quickly and leave you feeling more energized.

Vegan athletes have proven over and over that this diet and lifestyle not only sustains them but also helps them thrive. Take tennis stars Venus and Serena Williams. Venus became a vegetarian after she developed Sjögren's syndrome, an autoimmune illness that causes muscular pain and fatigue. The lifestyle eases Venus's symptoms. Serena went vegan to support her sister and, in 2013, won her fifth US Open title.

Even NFL players have gone vegan, like Arian Foster of the Houston Texans. *Men's Journal* magazine reported that four months after Foster announced his switch to a plant-based diet, he had gained "more yards on the field than nearly any other player in the NFL. By early November (2013), he had amassed 168 carries—for 659 yards—and nine touchdowns."[10]

The website Great Vegan Athletes (GreatVeganAthletes.com) contains inspirational story after inspirational story. The site annually names a Vegan Athlete of the Year, and in 2013 the award went to German strongman competitor Patrik Baboumian. A vegetarian since 2005 and a vegan since 2011, Baboumian has set world records in strongman events. Since 2009 he's held the log lift world record (under 105 kg division). He also won the Germany's Strongest Man title in 2011 by winning the open division at the German strongman nationals.

Many celebrities are also vegan and vegetarian. I'll bet you can recognize some of these names: Woody Harrelson, Natalie Portman, Lea Michele, Michelle Pfeiffer, Casey Affleck, Betty White, Alicia Silverstone, Ellen DeGeneres and Portia de Rossi, Olivia Wilde, Jessica Chastain, Russell Brand, Jenny McCarthy, Beyoncé and Jay Z, Johnny Depp, Brad Pitt, Toby Maguire, Sara Gilbert, Alec Baldwin, Russell Simmons, Joaquin Phoenix, Mike Tyson, Jared Leto, Paul McCartney, Ben Stiller, Forest Whitaker, Christina Applegate, and Pierce Brosnan.

---

10   Diane Vukovic, "Arian Foster: Profile of a Vegan NFL Star," PlenteousVeg, October 10, 2015, www.plenteousveg.com.

You may be thinking, all of this is fine for professionally trained athletes and celebrities with their own personal trainers and chefs, but what what about me you may ask? Can I really put this type of lifestyle in action and see the same types of benefits?

I say you can.

And one reason is that you and I live in a time when anywhere you go in the world, there are healthy choices available.

New York City: Setting the Trends for Healthy Living

In New York City, we have outstanding holistic doctors. They can help guide you to a healthier life and not just dispense medication if you have issues. If you live outside of New York, you can go to Happy Herbivore Plant-Based Doctors at HappyHerbivore.com to find the doctor that best suits your needs. For my fellow New Yorkers, here are some recommendations taken from the Happy Herbivore Plant-Based Doctors website:

- Dr. Ashutosh Tewari, surgeon and urologist, 625 Madison Ave., New York, NY 10022. (212) 241-9955.
- Dr. Elena Klimenko, doctor, internal medicine, 280 Madison Ave., #905, New York, NY 10016. (212) 696-4325.
- Dr. Ethan Ciment, podiatrist, 37 W. Twentieth St., New York, NY 10011. (646) 929-4149.
- Dr. James Borin, urologist, 150 E. Thirty-Second St., New York, NY 10016. (646) 825-6327.
- Dr. Martin Ehrlich, 245 Fifth Ave., New York, NY 10016. (646) 935-2252.
- Dr. Meghan Burke, pediatrician, 254 W. Eighty-Seventh St., New York, NY 10024. (212) 496-6440.
- Dr. Vincent M. Pedre III, 120 E. Fifty-Sixth St., Suite 530, New York, NY 10022. (212) 860-8300.
- Dr. Claudia Machado Cooke, alternative medicine, 35 E. Thirty-Fifth St., #206, New York, NY, 10016. (212) 213-0288.
- Dr. Frank Lipman, Eleven Eleven Wellness Center, 32 W. Twenty-Second St., Fifth Floor, New York, NY 10010. (212) 255-1800.
- Dr. Raphael Kellman, internist, the Kellman Center, 150 E. Fifty-Fifth St., Sixth Floor, New York, NY 10022. (212) 717-1118.

- Dr. Caroline Hartridge, osteopathy and general practitioner, 101 Hospital Rd., Patchogue, NY 11772. (704) 705-1481
- Dr. Michelle McMacken, internal medicine, 462 1ˢᵗ Ave., New York, NY 10016 (212) 562-1686.
- Dr. Robert Ostfeld, cardiologist, 3400 Bainbridge Ave., Bronx, NY 10467. (718) 920-5197.
- Dr. Carrie Bowler, osteopathic medicine, 794 Union St., Brooklyn, NY 11215. (212) 624-1077.
- Dr. Sapana Shah, internal medicine, 462 1ˢᵗ Ave., New York, NY 10016. (212) 562-1686

But maybe you personally feel at a loss about where to start. Sure, you can get a doctor who lays out a nutritional plan for you, but where do you shop? Where do you eat? How should you cook at home?

Actually, you are at a greater advantage than we have been in the past thanks to the vast world of the Internet. You can seek out whatever you need. When I went to plant-based eating, practically nobody else was doing it at the time. It was a very rare thing for someone not to eat meat. We didn't have the resources, the studies, and the wonderful vegetarian restaurants. There was no restaurant I could go to with friends. I used to get a baked potato and a side of broccoli when I went out to eat. Now you can go anywhere in the world and find vegetarian options anywhere, anytime—even before you step out of the door, as you can also have these healthy options delivered to you.

But today people are much more ready to recognize the health benefits of a vegetarian diet. Vegetarians don't just stop eating meat. By focusing on nutritious plants, fruits, and grains, they are automatically not eating a lot of processed foods and are embracing that idea with gusto.

If you were to take your own personal survey, you wouldn't believe the number of vegan and vegetarian restaurants in New York City. There's almost one on every block! We even have a vegan and vegetarian lunch truck and a vegan ice-cream truck. There are easy (and plentiful) ways for you to make the transition to this wonderful lifestyle. I'm sure there are similar options in your country, state, or town too.

If you are starting from scratch and still are unsure how to find this bounty of options, there's a website to help: HappyCow.net, which allows users to find, rate, and share their favorite places to eat. And it's not just limited to New York City—you can look up every area to find a vegan or vegetarian restaurant. Some cities have more options than others, obviously. For example, you can go to the Wynn in Las Vegas, which has a full vegetarian menu in every restaurant. And if you live in an area of the country where meat eating is more of the culture, HappyCow.net will still have a list. Try it out.

Another great resource is FriendsofAnimals.org, which produces a vegan-restaurant guide for New York City. You can download the current year's guide here: http://friendsofanimals.org/programs/veganism/vegan-restaurant-guides-and-reviews/new-york-vegan-restaurant-guide.

I also highly recommend *The Vegan Guide to New York City* by Rynn Berry and Max Friedman. It can be found on Amazon.com and has detailed reviews of more than 120 vegetarian and vegan restaurants, plus tips on where to find cheap organic produce, bulk grains, and exotic spices. The authors also tell you about cruelty-free and ecofriendly boutiques and stores.

As for me, here's a list of my favorite go-to places for great vegan and vegetarian fare.

For date night:

All of these restaurants make you feel welcome and special on date nights. They'll treat you like royalty!

- Hangawi: 12 E. Thirty-Second St., New York, NY 10016. (212) 213-0077. I've been going here for at least twenty years and find it magical!
- Candle 79: 154 E. Seventy-Ninth St., New York, NY 10075. (212) 537-7179. We also love this place, which has recently opened a second location on the Upper West Side.
- Blossom NYC: 187 Ninth Ave., New York, NY 10011. (212) 627-1144. Another location on the Upper West Side that is excellent is Blossom on Columbus: 507 Columbus Ave., New York, NY 10024. (212) 875-2600.
- Avant Garden: 130 E. Seventh St., New York, NY 10009. (646) 922-7948. The food is amazing and has become a new favorite spot to have a romantic dinner or bring our non vegan friends.
- Nix: 72 University Pl., New York, N.Y. 10003. (212) 498-9393. The food is seasonal, shareable and highly flavorful.
- Mother of Pearl: 95 Ave A, New York, NY 10009 (212) 614-6818. Postmodern Polynesian small plates and special cocktails and mock-tails. Fun atmosphere!
- Dirt Candy: 86 Allen St., New York, NY 10002 (212) 228-7732. Very different and a must try!

- Kajitsu: 125 East 39th St., New York, NY 10016 (212) 228-4873. Tranquil Japanese eatery for Kaiseki-style veggie meals.
- abcV: 38 East 19th St., New York, NY 10003 (212) 475-5829. Great seasonal plates, perfect for dinner or even brunch.
- Lady Bird: 111 E 17th St., New York, NY 10009 (917) 261-5524. A really fun atmosphere, Ladybird is a chic, trendy vegetable tapas restaurant.
- JaJaJa Plantas Mexicana: 162 E Broadway, New York, NY 10002 (646) 883-5453. A fun, contemporary Mexican spot with a colorful vegan menu.
- Delice & Sarrasin: 20 Christopher St., New York, NY 10014 (212) 243-7200. A quaint café offering traditional French dishes made vegan.
- PS Kitchen: 246 W 48th St., New York, NY 10036 (212) 651-7247. Breathtaking ambience and delicious food, the owner donates 100% of profits to sustainable charities locally and overseas.
- Bar Verde: 65 2nd Ave., New York, NY 10003 (212) 777-6965. Casual, contemporary vegan spot for tacos & other Mexican plates.
- Urban Vegan Kitchen: 41 Carmine St., New York, NY 10014 (646) 438-9939. Organic vegan comfort food.
- Modern Love: 317 Union Ave., Brooklyn, NY 11211 (929) 298-0626. Charming café serving elegant plates of vegan comfort food.

Personal note: It would not be fair to list these entire fantastic NYC vegetarian restaurants without including master chef Jay Astafa. While not having a permanent location as yet his pop up venues and catering for the many Vegan events in New York City are legendary. First expanding his family's pizzeria business on Long Island to include vegan options then opening his own vegan Italian restaurant in Copiague Long Island. Jay is clearly a rising star on a ever rising trend for this compassionate and delicious lifestyle.

I would also like to mention Pas Niratbhand who is the founder of "The Seed" which is a plant based Lifestyle Company. Pas is an amazing chef that also runs pop up culinary events at Exhibit C in Manhattan.

Less formal dinner or lunch:

- Terri: 60 West 23rd St, New York, NY 10010 (212) 647-8810. Second location is at 100 Maiden Ln., New York, NY 10038 (212) 742-7901.
- Blossom du Jour: Four locations. See BlossomduJour.com.

- Peacefood Café: Several locations. See www.peacefoodcafe.com/locations/.
- Beyond Sushi: 229 E. Fourteenth St., New York, NY 10003 (646) 861-2889. *Multiple locations
- Caravan of Dreams: 405 E. Sixth St., New York, NY 10009 (212) 254-1613.
- Jivamuktea Café: 841 Broadway, New York, NY 10003 (212) 353-0214.
- Candle Cafe West: 2427 Broadway, New York, NY 10024 (212) 769-8900.
- Mathew Kenney's Vegan Pizzeria 00 + Co.: 65 2nd Ave., New York, 10003 (212) 957-3005.
- Champs Diner: 197 Melrose St., Brooklyn NY 11206 (718) 599-2743. Vegan baked goods and comfort food served in retro diner.
- Go Zen: 144 W 4th St., New York, NY 10012 (212) 260-7130. Serving Asian cuisine in unique vegan small plates.
- VSPOT Organic: 12 St. Marks Place, New York, NY 10003 (212) 254-3693.
- by CHLOE: 185 Bleecker St., New York, NY 10012 (212) 290-8000.
  - Personal note: It would not be fair to list these entire fantastic NYC vegetarian restaurants without including master chef Jay Astafa. While not having a permanent location as yet his pop up venues and catering for the many Vegan events in New York City are legendary. First expanding his family's pizzeria business on Long Island to include vegan options then opening his own vegan Italian restaurant. Jay is clearing a rising star on a ever rising trend for this compassionate and delicious lifestyle. www.jayastafa.com (212) 858-9277
  - I would also like to mention Pas Niratbhand who is the founder of The Seed, which is a plant, based lifestyle company. Pas is an amazing chef that also runs pop ups at Exhibit C. www.theseedexperience.com (347) 474-0370

Power to the Power Smoothie!

I make a smoothie every day; because I strongly believe one meal a day should be liquid. First of all it gives my digestive system a needed rest. Plus I can add a lot of nutrients and vitamins and make one powerful drink to start my day. Smoothies are a big part of what I like to do and what I recommend to my clients. I also like smoothies over a juice in the morning, because juices remove the fiber that we need.

I use my Vitamix blender, which was a gift from my niece Dara, to make my smoothies. One other smoothie maker that is less expensive, which I also highly recommend, is NutriBullet.

Certain ingredients, like chia seeds, add fiber and help you to have beautiful poops and cleanse your system. Aloe juice is another ingredient that will cleanse your system if you add it to your smoothie.

Here's my suggested shopping list for basic ingredients to make an awesome smoothie:

- Powders: Sunwarrior protein powder, maca powder, green powder with advanced multivitamins
- Liquids: coconut milk, almond milk, soy milk, coconut yogurt (in place of regular yogurt if you're going vegan), chlorophyll with aloe vera juice
- Add-ins: chia seeds from Be Well probiotic powder, frozen organic fruits and veggies, nuts, hempseeds, flaxseeds, almond butter, greens; MCT oil from Be Well, by Dr. Frank Lipman (can be found at www.IreneRizzo.com)

And this is how I put it all together:

If you have a lot of things in your smoothie, you can pack a lot of nutrition into one sitting. Always include something green (meeting your chlorophyll requirement will ensure you're getting the vitamins your body needs). Smoothies are a great idea pre-workout to give you the energy you need and great post-workout to rebuild and restore you. They're good all the time.

And here's my secret for an awesome smoothie: I personally never measure anything. All the ingredients are so good, so your smoothie really just depends on what you like more. Do you like it sweeter? Throw in some dates. Thicker? Add chia seeds or a banana to it. One of the other things I tell clients is that if you don't have the ingredients in a standard smoothie recipe; take what you have in your house. If a quick survey of your refrigerator or pantry yields nothing, get creative with your staples on your grocery-shopping list so you will always have them available.

I tell my clients, don't make anything a big deal. Don't overthink it. If you have three things in your house—frozen organic vegetables, fruits, and nuts—then you have the basics for great smoothies.

As for me, I alternate ingredients depending on what I have on hand. But I always make sure I have frozen organic fruits and veggies in my freezer. They never go bad. And I try to freeze some bananas when they become too ripe. I always have them on hand.

I have been using nut and soy milk for a long time in my smoothies. However, I have discovered that most store-bought nut or soymilks have a lot of added ingredients. If it is a matter of convenience for you to buy your nut or soy milk instead of making it yourself, then you should. Just because something is labeled vegan or vegetarian, it does not mean it's healthy. Follow this rule of thumb when reading ingredient labels: if there are words you can't pronounce, it means it's not healthy. So read the labels!

But here's an easy recipe. Once you start making your own milk, you probably will never go back to store-bought!

My Nut and Coconut Milk Recipe

- Soak one cup of cashews or almonds in water overnight.
- The next morning, rinse with filtered water.
- Mix the nuts with Bob's Red Mill Date Crumbles to taste, depending on how sweet you like your milk (see BobsRedMill.com).
- Add a dash of vanilla.
- Blend on high speed with four cups of water.

If you prefer coconut milk, buy a Coco Jack (Coco-Jack.com), which is a tool for opening a coconut safely in seconds. Extract the coconut's meat, and follow the same recipe as you would for the nuts.

Smoothie Recipes

Here are some of my favorite smoothie recipes.

My Basic Recipe

Here's an easy shopping list of the ingredients you'll need:

- Sunwarrior protein powder (chocolate or vanilla)
- Chia seeds from Greens + Organics
- Be Well probiotic powder (available on IreneRizzo.com)
- Chlorophyll
- Aloe vera juice
- Maca powder

- Hempseeds
- Flaxseeds
- Almond, cashew, or walnut butter
- MCT oil from Be Well, by Dr. Frank Lipman
- Greens
- Green powder with advanced multivitamins
- Almond, cashew, or coconut milk

Here's how I put it all together:

Sunwarrior protein powder is a raw vegan protein that is gluten-free and soy-free, with a complete amino acid profile. I measure one scoop into my blender. I then throw in chia seeds and add from Be Well (available on my website) probiotic powder, chlorophyll with aloe vera juice, and maca powder.

Then I decide what I'm in the mood for that day. Sometimes I add hempseeds or flaxseeds. Sometimes I add almond butter. And sometimes I add MCT oil from Be Well, by Dr. Frank Lipman (by the way, his products are available on my website, IreneRizzo. com). I also use Greens Plus green powder with Advanced Multi. I usually make my own almond, cashew, or coconut milk. I also like to make smoothies out of kale, banana, pear, almond butter, and almond milk. They always come out consistently perfect. Another great smoothie is a combination of almond butter, almond milk, cacao nibs, and banana. And to top it off, I always add ice for me (no ice for my husband!). I measure to taste.

Green Pineapple Smoothie

- Super greens
- Cucumber
- Pineapple
- Spinach leaves
- Half an avocado
- Water
- Ice cubes
- Lime

Strawberry Oatmeal Smoothie

- Almond milk
- Baby oatmeal
- Banana
- Strawberries
- Vanilla protein powder

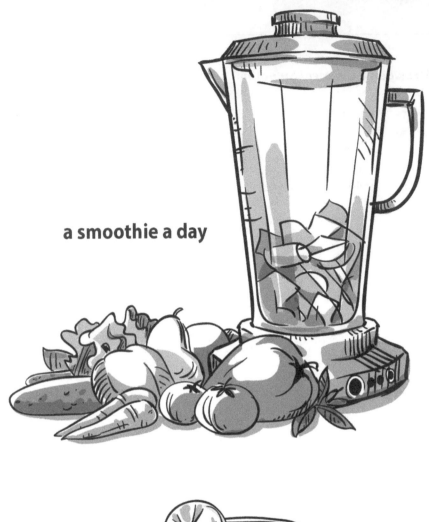

a smoothie a day

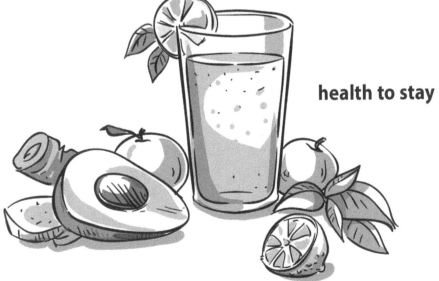

health to stay

My favorite smoothie to get in New York City is Terri's Vegan Café's green power smoothie, with almond milk instead of soy. You can make your own using, kale, pear, banana, almond butter and soy milk. I also love the joyful almond, with kale, at Juice Generation. Make your own using, almond butter, cacao nibs, banana, frozen, coconut milk, ice, and your choice of nut milk. I make it with dates instead of agave at home.

My favorite place for smoothies and juices is Juice Press. This place offers so many good ones! They make them fresh and replace agave nectar with dates. I'm not a big fan of agave nectar, which medical professionals have deemed far worse than high-fructose corn syrup.

Sometimes, during the colder months, I might not want a smoothie for my breakfast, so I like to make steel-cut oatmeal, and I have an easy method:

Put the called-for amount of steel-cut oatmeal and water according to the directions in your rice cooker or slow cooker. Leave it in overnight. The next morning you'll have perfect steel-cut oats every time!

Seven Days of Plant-Based Meals

Don't feel overwhelmed by a meal plan for a plant-based diet. This is what a seven-day meal plan looks like at my house:

Breakfast
Choice of:
Steel-cut oatmeal with fruit
Whole grain bread or millet and flax toast with walnut butter and jelly
Millet and flax muffin with avocado and tomatoes
I also recommend Sami's Bakery (SamisBakery.com), which makes excellent millet and flaxseed muffins.
Bob's Red Mill muesli with almond milk regular or vanilla
Smoothie (my weekday favorite!)
Vegan muffin with fruit
Sakara granola (SakaraLife.com) with coconut milk yogurt

Lunch
With any of these lunch entrees, add one to three of these delicious and nutritious side items: a sweet potato, rice, or a tossed salad.

Tofurky sandwich
Salad with Wildwood SprouTofu and nuts
Soup and salad
Hummus wrap
Veggie burger
Eggplant sandwich
Falafel pita
Almond butter and jelly sandwich
Best veggie dog: Field Roast

Dinner

Veggie stir-fry with Japanese sweet potatoes
Beans and rice with a side of broccoli
Zucchini pasta
Pasta
Veggie burrito
Veggie Italian or Mexican lasagna
Gardein Chick'n Scaloppini
Gardein Chipotle Black Bean Burger
Veggie pizza

Plant-Based Meal Recipes

Easy Black Beans & Rice

INGREDIENTS

FOR THE RICE:

- 1 cup organic brown rice
- 2 cups water or vegetable broth
- Himalayan salt to taste

FOR THE BEANS:

- 4 Tablespoons Cheeky Monkey Oil (more or less, taste preference)
- 1 onion finely diced
- 1 red pepper finely diced
- 1 zucchini diced
- 1 28-oz can of black beans, rinsed and drained
- Himalayan salt
- 1 cup water

INSTRUCTIONS

1. Cook rice, add salt to taste.
2. Meanwhile, for the beans; sauté onion, pepper, zucchini until all begin to brown.
3. Then add beans, water, salt; stir and simmer uncovered for at least 30 minutes, continue cooking until desired flavor is reached.

Delicious as a full meal or paired with a salad. I prefer to cook rice in a ricecooker, you can set in the morning and have it ready when you return home. I make the beans in my 360 cookware, I recommend their kitchen products to any health conscious cooks out there.

Zucchini Noodles

INGREDIENTS

- 4 Zucchinis
- 1 cup tomatoes
- 1cup cooked broccoli
- ½ cup vegetable broth
- 1 tablespoon olive oil

INSTRUCTIONS

1. Heat Use a vegetable peeler to cut slices off the zucchini lengthwise, stopping at the seeds. Then slice the flat strips into thin spaghetti strips.
2. Heat olive oil in skillet add garlic, zucchini strip, cook 1 minute, Add broth, tomatoes and broccoli, cook about 5 minutes, until zucchini has softened. Add salt and pepper to taste.

There are so many ways to make zucchini noodles, I like to top them with of my favorites: vegan pesto, tomato sauce, garlic and oil or a savory caper sauce. Get creative!

Roasted Cauliflower Head

INGREDIENTS

- Whole cauliflower head (remove center)
- Panko bread crumbs
- Mustard and/or Cheeky Monkey Oil
- Himalayan salt

INSTRUCTIONS

1. Preheat oven to 400. Brush cauliflower head with Cheeky Monkey Oil and/or mustard, next top with Panko breadcrumbs and salt.
2. Place cauliflower on a tray, cover in parchment paper then cover again with aluminum foil. Bake at least 1 hour, Cauliflower should look flaky.

Love Lasagna

INGREDIENTS

- 1 pot of Italian Tomato Sauce (about 5 cups)
- 1 pound uncooked lasagna noodles
- 1 ¾ cup Kite Hill vegan ricotta cheese
- 4 cups Miyoko's vegan mozzarella cheese
- ½ cup "Follow Your Heart" vegan parmesan cheese
- 1 pound bag organic carrots
- 1 bag raw organic spinach

INSTRUCTIONS

1. Prepare your favorite tomato sauce. Heat oven to 375.
2. Boil carrots then mash with potato masher.
3. Coat your baking pan with a little sauce. Add a layer of uncooked pasta, top with half of your vegan ricotta, add layer of ½ mashed carrots, then ½ raw spinach, top with ½ remaining sauce. Sprinkle on half of mozzarella.
4. Repeat with a layer of pasta, top with remaining ricotta, add remaining carrots and spinach, then another 1/3 of your sauce and the remaining mozzarella.
5. Add a layer of pasta, remaining sauce and top with vegan Parmesan.
6. Bake about 45 minutes, until melted and bubbly.
7. Let sit 5-10 minutes.

Vegan Substitute Guide.

Milk:

- Califia Farms
- Ripple

I prefer to create my own homemade nut milks, but these are excellent store bought varieties.

Creamer:

- Soy Delicious: Coconut creamer

Yogurt:

- Forager

Ice cream:

- Van Leeuwen
- Soy Delicious

Cream cheese:

- Kite hill

Riccotta cheese:

- Kite hill

Sour Cream:

- WayFare

American cheese:

- Follow Your Heart

White cheese slices

- Field Roast: Chao

Parmesan:

- Follow Your Heart

Mozzarella:

- Miyokos

Artisan Cheeses:

- Miyokos
- Riverdel Cheese

*VioLife: one of my favorite brands for all cheese varieties

Butter:

- Miyokos
- Earth balance

Mayo:

- Vegenaise

Tartar sauce:

- Follow Your Heart

Tofu:

- Hodo Soy tofu (ideal for tofu scrambles)
- Wildwood organic sprouted tofu

Egg Substitutes for Baking:

- Follow Your Heart egg replacer
- Applesauce
- Mashed bananas
- Arrowroot powder
- Chia seed
- "Flegg" made from milled Flaxseed

Meat Substitutes:

- Beyond Meat Burger
- Gardein Meatballs
- Gardein Crab Cakes
- Gardein Turkey Roast
- Field Roast Frankfuters
- Field Roast Italian sausage

*When it comes to meat substitutes, Gardein is a great brand across the board.

The Compassionate Life

My closing thoughts to you are:

Be more conscious of where your food comes from.

Healthy eating leads to compassionate thinking and vice versa.

Today, following a vegan or vegetarian lifestyle is easier than ever.

One can only hope that in the future, animal abuse will stop, and people will realize how strong the health benefits are of a plant-based lifestyle. I do believe that eventually everyone will follow a plant-based diet. We don't need to hunt for our food in a civilized society. We have the availability of natural food that is delicious, and vegetables have everything we need in them. My hope for humanity is that everyone will eventually embrace a plant-based lifestyle. Can this end world hunger? Research tends to lean this way. Can it save the planet? Most likely, yes. Animals are living creatures, just like we are. The only difference between animals being used for industry and horrific historical crimes against humanity is the species. Think about it.

My hope is that this book will show you how to become healthier than you ever imagined—and in the process of employing healthy lifestyle decisions that honor all living creatures on this planet, you'll watch your compassionate heart flourish. That, in turn, will lead you on to a level of enlightenment that allows you to fully embrace all the beauty and joy that this planet and life of ours has to offer.

Questions

Learn from yesterday, live for today, hope for tomorrow.
The important thing is not to stop questioning.
—ALBERT EINSTEIN

Questions wake people up. They prompt new ideas.
They show people new places and new ways of doing things.

—MICHAEL MARQUARDT

Some questions are more important than the answers.
—NANCY WILLARD

1. Does Pilates make you taller?

Since Pilates emphasizes strengthening and stretching your muscles, it helps correct posture by improving alignment. This allows you to reverse any damage or natural shrinkage (which occurs over time due to spinal discs compressing). It does not, however, lengthen your bones. Pilates teaches you how to articulate and lengthen your spine, making you stand and sit taller.

2. Tucking versus neutral spine—which one is more beneficial?

When I first start working with clients, I find that most people want to tuck their pelvises during various exercises. Sometimes people's bodies actually remain in a tucked-pelvis position throughout their lives, whether they are standing, sitting, or lying down. It's what they've become accustomed to and what feels normal. They think they are protecting their backs, yet they are hurting themselves.

Years ago, when I first started teaching, this was considered the right way. Research has shown that a neutral pelvis (which is keeping the natural curves in your spine) is more beneficial to the safety of your body. Tucking and squeezing and using your hip flexors instead of using your abdomen will compress the spine, and that is what you want to avoid. By working in neutral, you are working with the natural curves of your spine.

3. What are weight-bearing exercises?
Walking, jogging, dance, aerobics, hiking, weights, yoga, climbing stairs, tennis, and Pilates. Swimming and biking are not weight-bearing but are good exercises to maintain your weight and heart health (the best exercises for your bones are exercises that force you to work against gravity).

4. How much exercise is needed to maintain bone health?
Thirty minutes three to four times a week at minimum.

5. How much exercise is needed for weight loss?
Remember the 80/20 rules: 80 percent is diet, and 20 percent is exercise. When it comes to weight loss, exercise needs to become a daily habit for at least sixty minutes a day five to six days a week.

6. Is too much exercise harmful?
Yes. Extreme exercise, especially in young competitive athletes, can lead to decreased bone density, and overdoing it can lead to many different injuries, since it wears down the bones and does not allow time to rest and rebuild.

7. Can I spot reduce my body?
No! The concept of spot reduction follows the false belief that training a specific muscle will result in fat loss in that area of the body. The body works together as one. If you are lean already, you can get more muscle tone in that area, but if you are trying to lose weight in a specific area, you need do fat-burning exercises, such as walking, running, biking, tennis, Pilates, or yoga (or choose your favorite full-body activity). Full-body exercises will assist in overall weight loss. Remember, 80 percent is diet, and 20 percent is exercise.

8. Why does my midsection expand as I get older, and how can I reduce it?
Well, there are a few reasons why fat starts to accumulate in the stomach area as we age. For women it can be the reality of menopause. Menopause causes a loss of

estrogen, and this makes a recipe for more fat cells. Also, progesterone levels tend to slow, causing bloating and water-weight gain. But there are a variety of reasons that both men and woman experience midsection expansion: genetic predisposition, poor diet, and lack of exercise, to name a few. Women compared to men are actually less prone to belly fat, but as we age, our metabolisms slow, and our hormones change, even our distribution of fat changes—our legs, arms, and hips get smaller and our bellies larger.

The best way to try to reduce belly fat is to eat a healthy diet rich in fruits, vegetables, and whole grains along with proper hydration. My best suggestion, along with the above, is to avoid eating anything out of a box, bag, or can to reduce or eliminate additives and unnecessary sugars. And, of course, create a daily routine of moderate to intense cardio activity, a minimum of thirty minutes a day. Exercise reduces stress, and stress can be a big factor in the accumulation of belly fat. Exercise will decrease cortisol levels and aid in the reduction of belly fat.

Here's a special note for women who have been pregnant and are having difficulty reducing their belly bulges regardless of any exercise or diet they have attempted: You may be experiencing a tear in the abdominal wall. It is called *rectus diastasis*. Certain exercises can assist in strengthening this muscle, and in extreme cases surgery is needed; either way, your healing can begin, and your weight loss can be attained.

9. Should I feel the burn when exercising?
The burn really means there is a buildup of lactic acid, which can be described as an achy, burning sensation your muscles feel after doing intense exercise. Your body is telling you the lactic acid is building up. Some people feel this is a sign that your body is working up to potential and that you will see results, hence the phrase "feel the burn." However, while the burn can be seen as a sign that you have worked your body out hard and can feel the triumph, it can also be a sign of danger. When exercises are not properly done or an incorrect form is taking place, you can still feel the burn, but injury may be lurking just around the corner. In other words, the burn can be misleading. The solution is to exercise safely; pick a routine that is reasonable for your fitness level, and the goal should be to strengthen your muscles using great form. Don't let the burn tell you what is and what isn't working.

10. What can I do so my neck doesn't hurt while doing abdominal exercises?
If you put your hands behind your neck, do not pull on it. Feel the weight of your head in your hands, and then nod your head forward, like you're holding a tennis ball between your chin and chest. Make sure your stomach muscles bring you up. Do this slowly—no

pulling. Once you learn this, you can build up to hands-free. Remember, if you feel a strain, keep your head down. Also, you can start from a seated position and roll down holding behind your legs, keeping your neck free.

11. Should I use an exercise tracker?
Exercise trackers are great self-motivators. Some of the many benefits of various trackers include calculating your steps; evaluating your sleep patterns; measuring you water intake; and, if you're looking for a competitive edge, involving your friends in a step challenge, which can add to your motivation. I recommend and prefer using the tracker built in to a phone. I also like the benefit of having my personal information on my phone in case of an emergency, and it makes my walks more relaxed knowing communication is a few taps away.

12. What about the latest exercise trends? Are they worth trying?
I do have to say that some trendy exercises can be a fun break in routine, but they don't always last. That's why they are called trends. With that said, I believe sticking with forms of exercise that have lasted through the years, like Pilates, yoga, and walking, might just be your best choice.

13. Why are balance exercises so important—even more so as we age?
Poor balance can cause falls, especially in older adults. These falls can be serious and even life threatening. The more you practice, the better your balance becomes. It's best to start practicing balance early in life, but you're never too old to start. Balance can be as simple as standing on one leg for as little as five seconds and working up to a minute or so or as challenging as standing on a BOSU ball.

14. What can I do about tight muscles?
I always recommend warming up your muscles before you stretch them, using heat, active exercise, a brisk walk, or marching in place. Two of my favorite solutions are foam rolling (you can purchase a foam roller at BalanceBody.com, and look for my how-to video on YouTube) and using a tennis ball to work out any tightness.

15. How do I avoid leg cramps?
Check your magnesium and potassium levels, and make sure you are hydrated.

16. What makes bones stronger?
Exercise weekly focused on weight-bearing routines. It makes the bones grow stronger and helps maintain bone mass.

17. How do I increase my bone density if I'm not taking calcium supplements?
Eat green leafy vegetables (e.g., kale, broccoli). Eat beans, and do weight-bearing exercises. Drinking milk does not improve bone integrity.

18. What else is necessary to maintain bone health?
A proper diet!

19. Is it OK to salt my food or eat foods containing salt? How much is too much?
If you choose an unrefined salt that is rich in trace minerals and free of additives, such as pink Himalayan salt (which is the only salt I use), then yes, it is OK to salt your foods. Subjects consuming less than 2,300 milligrams of sodium per day had a significantly higher mortality rate than others consuming 2,300 milligrams or more per day. Salt aids in blood-sugar control by improving insulin sensitivity, and it is a natural antihistamine. Your body also needs salt to maintain proper stomach pH. Salt lowers adrenaline spikes, improves sleep quality, aids in maintaining a healthy weight balance, supports thyroid function, and balances hormones—and it tastes good. So if you are not dealing with high blood-pressure issues (check with your doctor) and it's unrefined, salt away.

20. What are the benefits of vitamin E?
Vitamin E is key for strong immunity and healthy skin and eyes. In recent years vitamin E supplements have become popular as antioxidants. These are substances that protect cells from damage. Dosing for vitamin E can be confusing, so I suggest you look up dosing on WebMD or consult a doctor or a nutritionist. I personally prefer to get my vitamin E from food.

21. What foods are rich in vitamin E?
Green leafy vegetables, such as spinach and broccoli; sunflower seeds; almonds; whole grains; carrots; nuts; wheat germ; avocados; squash such as pumpkin, butternut, and zucchini; kiwi; olive oil; cereals; and certain health breads.

22. What fats can I eat, and which ones should I avoid to maintain a healthy diet?
All fats have the same amount of calories, but they vary in their chemical compositions and effects on health.

List of Healthy Fats
Eating healthy fats in moderation fulfills your dietary fat needs without increasing your chronic disease risks. Examples of heart-healthy fats include plant-based oils, such as olive, walnut, soybean, and flaxseed; nuts; seeds; nut butters; avocados; and olives. Nuts and seeds are rich in heart-healthy fats as well as fiber and protein, which increase satiety, so they are an ideal choice when eating in small portions.

Fats to Avoid
Bad fats are those that increase your chronic disease risk when consumed in excess. These include saturated animal fats found in butter, lard, whole milk, ice cream, cream, cheese, and high-fat meats like bacon. Plant-based fats that have been hydrogenated and contain trans fats—found in margarines, shortenings, fried foods, and commercially baked goods—also increase your risk for heart disease, so avoid them.

23. If I am not eating meat, where can I get my protein?
I haven't eaten meat for forty-eight years. I have never worried about where I would get my protein. There is protein in everything—beans, grains, and vegetables such as broccoli, where 49 percent of the calories are protein. If you are worried and want to add extra protein, you can always use a natural vegan protein powder like Sunwarrior to your morning smoothie. But if you are eating a variety of foods, you will attain the protein your body needs.

24. What is the difference between steel-cut and pre-rolled oats?
Some may think all oats are created equal, but that is just not true. The difference lies in the amount of processing they endure. Steel-cut oats are not processed; they are left raw, while rolled oats are squeezed through a roller and steamed. Steel-cut is chewier and nuttier; rolled is precooked, has a mushy texture, and lacks the nutty flavor. And, of course, sugary packaged instant oats are low on the nutritional chain and are not a healthy choice, as they have added sugar you

don't need. Leave it on the shelf. (See my overnight oatmeal recipe in the previous chapter.)

25. Should I eat six small meals or three meals a day?
There are no established studies to say which is more beneficial. There are pros and cons to both, so it makes sense to find which one works best for you and what makes you feel good. Six meals a day keeps your metabolism going at a steady rate, which is great, but the benefits to three meals is your body gets a chance to digest each meal before you go on to the next. So make a choice you can stick with.

26. Should I eat breakfast?
Yes! I find a great deal of my clients who have weight issues tend to skip breakfast, which is not helpful to the body. Eating a healthy breakfast that is not high in sugar and fat (see my healthy breakfast list earlier in this book) will kick-start your metabolism and give you the energy to start your day. It is also known that people who skip breakfast tend to eat more calories throughout the day. So eat your breakfast.

27. I'm confused about soy. Is it good for you or not?
Yes, it is, but it depends on the kind of soy you are consuming. Fermented soy is best; sprouted and organic are also great sources, such as tofu and edamame. Whatever form you choose, it is best to make sure it is organic! I was brought up on soy, and I raised my own children on it. I have read all the studies, both the pros and cons, and the benefits outweigh the risks. Basically, it is a wonderful source of protein, and it is a much healthier choice than consuming red meat.

28. How obsessed should I be about my calorie intake?
I have abandoned calorie counting. Calories do count, but if you eliminate processed foods, reduce animal protein, avoid dairy, and don't eat too many times a day or too late, there is no need to worry about them.

29. How can I keep food fresh?
I recommend Fresh and Vital (ChiEnergyProducts.com). It's a card you place in your refrigerator, and it increases the shelf life of food, keeps food fresh, and saves money. It is environmentally safe and friendly and energizes your food.
    There is also an FDA storage chart (FDA.gov) that will tell you how long something will keep in the refrigerator or freezer.

30. Is coffee good for me?

There are definitely pros and cons. If you must have it, make sure it is organic. Remember, the caffeine in coffee is a drug, and anything you must have can't be good for you. It has been proven that the caffeine in coffee helps relieve headaches, improves memory, and aids diabetes, but if you feel you have to drink it or you can't do without it, it becomes an addiction. Remember, everything in moderation is always the rule for balanced health. So if you're going to drink up, stick to one cup a day that is organic and not filled with artificial sweeteners and creamers.

31. I'm allergic to dairy, so I started drinking almond milk but found I had the same reaction. If I eat almonds, I don't have any symptoms. What's happening?

You have to look at all the ingredients in everything you eat. Sometimes an ingredient can be found in many different products. In the case of almond milk versus cow milk, an ingredient called casein may be added, which many are sensitive to. It is an added chemical that can never be good for your body. Make sure the form of milk you are drinking is pure.

32. What is casein?

It is the main protein in milk and in cheese (in the coagulated form). It is used in processed foods and in adhesive, paints, and other industrial products.

33. What makes wine vegan?

Even though wine is made from grapes, it also may have been made using animal-derived products, like blood, bone marrow, casein (milk protein), and chitin (fiber from crustacean shells). I will avoid boring you with the long, detailed process of how wine is made and what its contents may be; it is best to search out vegan wine distributers and choose your favorite. Know that you will avoid headaches, nausea, and possible hangovers with an organic vegan wine not only because it is devoid of chemicals but also because it's minus various animal-derived products. It can also bring you joy knowing no animal suffered for your wine pleasure. Again, everything in moderation; this does not mean you should go out and consume several bottles of wine in one sitting. Sip slowly and enjoy. And remember, for every glass of wine you consume, drink a glass of water.

34. How do I know which beauty products are safe for me and not tested on animals?

I recommend the Cruelty Cutter app and the PETA and Humane Society websites, which have lists of products. The Leaping Bunny (LeapingBunny.org) also connects compassionate consumers with cruelty-free companies. I use and recommend Tata

Harper and 100% Pure; they are animal safe and two of my favorites, but there are many other good products out there.

35. What cookware do you recommend?

I recommend and use 360 cookware. Some of its benefits are superior stainless steel and healthier cooking technology. It retains vitamins and nutrients; it's easy to clean—no need to use oil, only to taste; and it is made in America. I also like and use Le Creuset, which is a combination of cast iron and stainless steel—a safer way to prepare food. You don't want to cook with aluminum or nonstick cookware, as it is not worth the health risk. Dr. Barnard, who lost both parents to Parkinson's disease and has done research on the brain, feels that Parkinson's and Alzheimer's diseases are both caused by the buildup of metals in the brain over time. When they reach a toxic level, they release free radicals, which attack your brain cells.

36. What do you recommend for constipation?

If your diet consists of vegetables and fruits, you won't have to deal with constipation, but if you do, I recommend aloe juice in your smoothie or aloe with a little apple juice. Castor oil works miracles as well. Also try Calm (NaturalVitality.com) and Smooth Move by Traditional Medicinals (TraditionalMedicinals.com).

37. What can I do to clear my mind?

Meditation is the best way to clear your mind from the day's clutter or as a midafternoon refresher. Spiritual leaders like Deepak Chopra offer meditation programs, as does Louise Hay. In a pinch you can use a meditation application such as Simple Being, which offers five- to forty-five-minute meditations or an endless loop along with a sound of your choice (ocean, birds, light rain, and more). The app can be purchased on iTunes.

38. What can I do for colds and sore throats?

The following have always worked for my family and me: zinc and vitamin C, Power Pak Electrolyte Stamina and Immune Support Drink (which can be found on Amazon. com), Throat Coat, Gypsy Cold Care, and Breathe Easy.

39. What are your top tips for weight loss?

My 5 top tips are:

Write everything down, drink at least half your body weight in ounces daily, chew your food, exercise, and eat lots of fruits and vegetables.

40. Can dogs be vegan?
Yes, absolutely. My small dog has been vegan most of his life and is now thirteen. We also rescued a Doberman who lived most of her life as a vegan and died at fourteen years old. Dobermans are known to have heart issues and a life span of nine to eleven years. I think this says a lot about how a plant-based diet can affect longevity in animals.

There are several brands of vegan foods available. The one I currently use is Wysong; it is a dry wholesome food while Nature's Recipe makes a terrific vegan stew. Natural Balance and V-Dog are another brands that make vegan food for dogs as well as Pet Guard, which is also totally organic.

The pet food industry as a whole is a large consumer of animal products, and it is much less regulated than producing food for human consumption. By now you can connect the dots; there is no need for more industries supporting animal suffering when there are alternatives that are better. I am encouraged to see food choices available for our pets because as you now know, our four legged friends will thrive as vegans!

41. Are all your shoes, coats and handbags Vegan Too?
Now they are. For me it was a fast transition aligning with my commitment to this lifestyle, but transition for most people accelerates as they learn about and experience offerings that are made without animals being part of the business model. Whether it is for medical testing or the need to use their skin to make products, breeding and slaughtering animals for business at the end of the day is cruel. The choice is yours to become acquainted with the products and designers that support this way of thinking.

I have never had to go without great shoes and neither has my husband. I love fashion. Here are just a few of my favorite designers: Stella McCarrtney and Leanne Mai-ly Higart of Vaute Couture (I have a ton of her coats). For men the standout designer is Joshua Katcher of The Brave Gentle Man.

See my shopping list of great stores and websites that feature either completely or offer great options that are Vegan.

Vegan Fashion Shopping List

Vegan designers and brands

- **VAUTE** COUTURE. Stylish and warm outerwear, dresses, shirts, and jewelry. Visit the New flagship store in New York. 114 Stanton Street NYC.
- **Love is Mighty**. Gorgeous vegan shoes combining old-world textiles with modern designs
- **Brave Gentle Man**. NYC-based all-vegan attire, shoes, accessories, and custom suits www.bravegentleman.com
- **MATT & NAT**. Design-centric, eco-friendly and vegan handbags and accessories
- **Susan Nichole**. Vegan handbags, wallets, and more
- **Gunas.** 100% cruelty-free eco-friendly bags
- **OlsenHaus**. Pure vegan boots, wedges, flats, and more
- **Cri de Coeur**. Ethical contemporary shoes, handbags, and jewelry
- **Beyond Skin**. Designer non-leather women's shoes
- **Pansy Maiden**. Fashion-forward, cruelty-free bags and clutches
- **Neuaura**. Unique animal-free and eco-friendly footwear
- **Mammouth Outerwear Functional,** stylish vegan parkas and bombers
- **Melie Bianco**. Stylish, luxurious, animal-friendly handbags at an affordable price

- **NOAH**. Italian vegan shoes, famous worldwide for quality and comfort
- **Deux Lux**. Women's fashion handbags and accessories; glamorous, edgy, and ethical
- **Cornelia Guest.** Cruelty-free designer handbags.
- **John Bartlett**. Be sure to check out the Ambassador Collection, which supports Farm Sanctuary
- **Novacas**. Animal-friendly, environmentally-friendly, and worker-friendly shoes for men and women
- **Vegetarian Shoes**. Featuring leather-free shoes, hiking boots, and belts
- **NOHARM**. Offering vegan shoes, boots, accessories, and clothing
- **Lookie Lou**. An online vegan boutique that carries a carefully curated collection of ethically produced women's apparel and accessories
- **Mohop**. Hand-made vegan shoes with interchangeable ribbons for thousands of styles
- **Big Buddha**. Eye-catching bags made from vegan "V-Leather"
- **Freedom of Animals** A line of sustainable and cruelty-free luxury bags
- **Delikate Rayne** Cruelty-free women's contemporary luxury
- **Bead and Reel** A vegan owned online boutique carrying over 40 ethical designers
- **Jill Milan** Entirely vegan brand offering handbags and coats.
- **Saved Kisses** Soft, comfortable, cruelty-free and sustainable clothing line

Companies offering vegan products

- **Stella McCartney**. Womens ready to wear, Mostly vegan-friendly clothing and lingerie, always fur- and leather-free
- **Steve Madden/Madden Girl**. Many non-leather styles available
- **LuLu*s**. Online boutique with an entire section dedicated to vegan shoes
- **H&M**. Department store with vegan bags, shoes, and accessories galore
- **Forever 21**. Browse their collection for faux-leather boots, belts, hats, and more
- **Charlotte Russe**. Everything from faux snake-skin pumps to wool-free pea coat
- **Patagonia**. Look for parkas stuffed with PrimaLoft®, a super-warm down alternative

- **Zappos**. Just type "vegan" into the search bar of this online shoe store for endless selection.
- **Blowfish.** Edgy-cool footwear with the trendsetter in mind.
- **Melissa** Tech savvy footwear company
- **Anton Ello** Eco conscious handbags

One-stop shopping

Don't miss these 100% vegan online retailers, who carry many of the brands listed above, plus many more!

- **BraveGentleMan.com**
- **MooShoes.com** (visit the NYC storefront at 78 Orchard!)
- **AlternativeOutfitters.com**
- **CompassionCoutureShop.com**
- **VeganChic.com**
- **VeganStore.com**
- **VeganEssentials.com**
- **VeganEtsy.com**
- **VeganScene**

Vegan fashion tips

- **GirlieGirlArmy.com**. The Glamazon Guide to Conscious Living
- **TheDiscerningBrute.com**. Fashion, food, and etiquette for the ethically handsome man

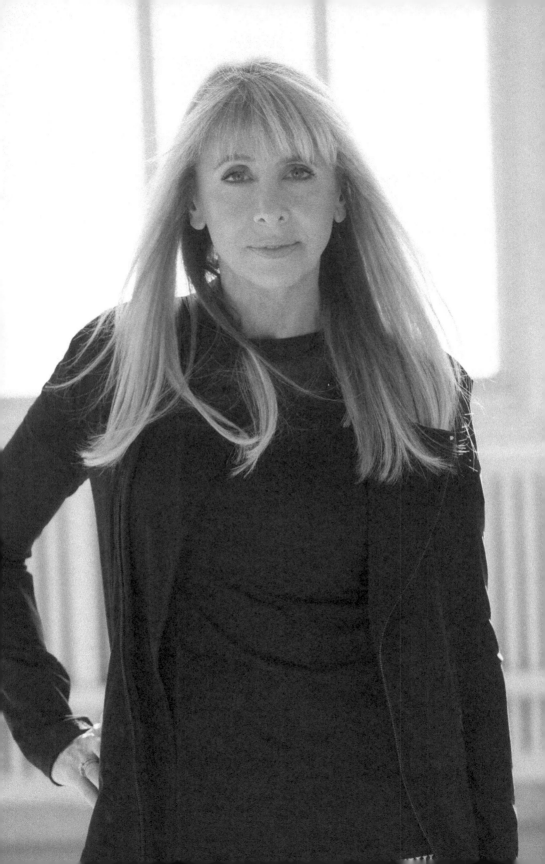

Author's Note

A journey of a thousand miles begins with one step.
—LAO TZU

wish you all the passion you could conjure up inside as you find fitness and discover your personal Mountain of Youth. I hope my book and the information have inspired you to make healthy changes. Set out for a new beginning. I know you can do it. Use the tools and information to start, and stay focused on the life you have been longing for, one filled with new energy, strength, and wellness—one that will catapult you into living your dreams of a long vibrant life.

I am here if you need me via the Internet. IreneRizzo.com, and my Facebook page. There will be messages, exercise tips and demonstrations, recipes, and more on Instagram and YouTube. You can also send me questions, and I will do my best to answer them.

Remember to be kind and loving to yourself and all living things. Think positively, and keep climbing your own personal Mountain of Youth!

Ending note: If you are curious about factory farming please plan a visit to a farm sanctuary and they will put it into focus. Farm Sanctuaries are a wonderful family outing and serve not only as a rescue for animals but they also provide education, lobbying and a window into the world of how animals would choose to live it they were free on a farm.

In New York State here are incredible sanctuaries I recommend to visit:

1. Farm Sanctuary, Watkins Glen NY, Orland CA, Los Angeles CA, and New Jersey
2. Woodstock Farm Sanctuary, High Falls NY
3. Catskill Animal Sanctuary, Saugerties NY